HPS Blanco

Paris 27-Febrero 79.

BRACHYTHERAPY

BRACHYTHERAPY

BERNARD PIERQUIN, M.D.
Professor of Radiotherapy
Hopital Henri Mondor
Creteil (Val-de-Marne), France

DANIEL J. CHASSAGNE, M.D.
Professor of Radiology
Institut Gustave-Roussy
Villejuif (Val-de-Marne), France

CHAHIN M. CHAHBAZIAN, M.D.
Associate Clinical Professor of Radiology
University of California at Irvine
Irvine, California

J. FRANK WILSON, M.D.
Assistant Professor of Radiology
Medical College of Wisconsin
Milwaukee, Wisconsin

WARREN H. GREEN, INC.
St. Louis, Missouri, U.S.A.

Published by

WARREN H. GREEN, INC.
8356 Olive Boulevard
St. Louis, Missouri 63132, U.S.A.

Library of Congress Catalog Card No. 72-117614
ISBN No. 0-87527-164-2

Printed in the United States of America

FOREWORD

In the beginning, all therapeutic applications of radioactive materials fell into what we designate today as *brachytherapy.* It was only later, when sufficient amounts of radium became available for irradiation at distances of a few centimeters away from the tumor, that Forssell (1931) proposed the terms brachytherapy and teletherapy to emphasize the difference. The term *Plesiotherapy,* proposed by Perussia (1948), was also used for short-range irradiation.

The earliest therapeutic trials carried on in Paris by Danlos with 150 milligrams of radium loaned by Pierre Curie, incorporated the radium salt into a sort of water-repellent varnish; it was painted on a variety of applicators of various shapes, mostly for surface and intracavitary irradiation (1904). Radium was also used for interstitial implantation: Abbé of New York (1905) placed celluloid tubes within tumors and used them later to introduce removable radium sources. The came the therapeutic utilization of *radon.* At first the vials containing the radioactive radium emanation were brought into contact with the surface of tumors. Duane of Boston perfected a radon extraction plant (1915) and conceived the idea of concentrating the short-life radioactive gas into capillary tubes that were easily segmented, implanted into tumors and left to decay. Duane's bare "glass seeds" administered unfiltered radiations. Regaud and Debièrne (1915) of Paris placed the capillary glass tubes containing radon in Platinum sheaths for interstitial implantation and removal. Failla (1926) substituted capillary gold tubes for glass and originated the "gold seeds," continuing to favor the abandonment of sources to decay within the tissues.

The early practice of brachytherapy brought to light the possibilities of success as well as the complications and reasons for failure. It became evident that to be eligible for this approach, amenable tumors had to be *accessible,* and geometrically *delimitable* and of *moderate size.* The inherent characteristics of these modalities were unavoidable: *continous irradiation* at a *low hourly rate* but a rather *intensive total dose* delivered in a short number of days. Practiced on a much greater scale at first, the indications for radium therapy gradually decreased with the development of high voltage roentgentherapy and cobalt 60 teletherapy. However, some of these applications have remained with us throughout the years as useful adjuvants of surgery or other radiotherapeutic approaches: intracavitary vaginal and uterine irradiation as a complement of external pelvic irradiation, interstitial irradiation of primary carcinomas of the lateral border of the tongue.

The development of artificial radioactivity has brought us a richer armamentarium,new sources capable of being fashioned in accomodating ways. The new radiation emitters can be utilized in better ways, and the pragmatic development of after-loading has made the procedures safer for the medical personnel and more accurate for the patients. Thus is explained the greater sophistication and resurgence of interest in brachytherapy exemplified by this volume.

Bernard Pierquin, heir of one of the pioneers of the Foundation Curie, himself a former member of the staff of the Institut Roussy of Paris, has become identified in the development of present techniques of brachytherapy. Highly dedicated, he has persistently applied himself to the development of intrumentation and techniques as well as organization that are required for better results. Pierquin has honed the procedures and sharpened the didactics to allow a greater number of radiotherapists to undertake these procedures. With his associate and successor, Daniel J. Chassagne, he has made useful additions to the medical literature on the subjet of utilization of brachytherapy.

The original French version of this book often adopted the style, well known to French medical audiences, of the *cahiers de l'internat.* This English version represents an important revision of the original text; in addition, it is presented in the customary medical narrative. My former associates, C.M. Chahbazian and J. Frank Wilson, together with D. J. Chassagne have labored to bring forth an English version of this work, which can be recognized as the clearest guide and up-to-date information on the subject of brachytherapy. Indeed, this revised text is now to be considered for publication as a new French version. A profusion of diagrams contributes to the didactic endeavor of the authors; additional references given facilitate the extension of information and details.

Because of my long professional acquaintance with the authors and translators of this work as well as in recognition of the excellence of their work, I am honored to have been asked to write this foreword and pleased to present this English version to radiotherapists everywhere.

J. A. del Regato, M.D.
Professor of Radiology
University of South Florida College of Medicine

INTRODUCTION

Since the publication of our *Precis de Curietherapie* in 1964 (1), the techniques and results of brachytherapy have become better defined. In 1977, we can establish more precisely and selectively the methods and the therapeutic indications of this nascent branch of radiotherapy.

In photon or gamma therapy, in accordance with the recommendations of the International Atomic Energy Agency (2), only two sealed radioactive elements have been retained; namely, Cesium 137 and Iridium 192. The other radioactive elements, whether artificial isotopes such as Cobalt 60, Tantalum 182, or Gold 198 or natural isotopes such as Radon 222 or Radium 226, can now be eliminated from current practice and assume their place in the museum of brachytherapy.

The selective choice of these two elements is based upon their adaptability to afterloading (3), an indispensible condition of precise and controlled application of the sources. Afterloading implies the meticulous insertion or implantation of nonradioactive supporting or guide hardware which is later quickly loaded with or replaced by radioactive sources. Sources must meet four basic technical requirements in afterloading:

1. **Miniaturization** — a sufficient amount of radioactive material must be miniaturized so that it can be introduced into carrier systems. This implies procurement of wires, needles or seeds less than 0.7 mm in diameter.

2. **Pliability** — the material should meet the requirements of both strength and maleability. One should be able to adapt this material with safety to all anatomopathological conditions.

3. **Adequate protection** in conformity with the required regulations (4) which implies three conditions:

a. **The source** must be perfectly sealed in order to eliminate any radioactive contamination of the facilities or personnel.

b. **Containers** must be lightweight and easily transportable imposing the choice of low energy gamma emitters.

c. **The application** of the radioactive sources should be completed as rapidly as possible with the help of remote control emphasizing again the afterloading technique.

4. **A resonable cost** of radioactive sources either in the form of relatively short-lived, low energy emitters with a high degree of efficiency such as Iridium 192 or in the form of long half-life emitters such as Cesium 137.

In electron or beta therapy, three sealed pure beta emitters have been retained namely Phosphorus 32 in plastic applicators, Strontium 90 in metallic applicators essentially making use of the secondary radiations of its daughter element Yttrium 90, which can itself also be used either as free-form seeds or as needles.

This profound evolution of brachytherapy since 1964 has led us to publish an entirely new book in 1977 and to make its English translation available. The text and illustrations of the new work are mostly original to make their adaptation to current understanding of this subject more complete.

I would like to draw the reader's attention to the place of brachytherapy in the general specialty of radiation therapy by emphasizing the terminology and the responsibility of the brachytherapist. Presently the terminology of radiation therapy is rather confusing. It would be very desirable to finally agree upon a few key words, especially in the two international languages of English and French. We propose to subdivide radiation therapy into two main branches; namely, teletherapy and brachytherapy.

Teletherapy applies to all techniques using radioactive sources at a distance of more than 5 cm from the tumor, irrespective of the energy and the characteristics of the radiation.

Brachytherapy applies to all techniques using radioactive sources at less than 5 cm distance from, or inside the tumor, Plesiotherapy referring to radioactive sources close to the tumor, and Endotherapy to when they are imbedded within the tumor.

The responsiblity of the brachytherapist deserves a comment. His role, as in all radiotherapeutic applications, is to obtain a homogeneous and adequate distribution of the dose so that the reference isodose, upon which the tumor dose is calculated, coincides with the boundaries of the volume to be irradiated, while keeping the dose to the surrounding normal tissues at a mimimum. The brachytherapist should be capable of controlling the dose at any point in the radioactive application. This role requires great competence and long experience in dosimetry and radiology learned through many years of training. He should also acquire surgical skill of sufficient degree to enable him to apply the radioactive sources safely, with his own hands, under aseptic conditions. In fact, we cannot dissociate the responsibility of the surgical act from that of its radiological consequences.

Finally, I would like to extend my gratitude to all who helped in the preparation of the work. First of all, I am indebted to Daniel Chassagne who was my first student and who succeeded me as chief of the Department of Curietherapy at Institut Gustave Roussy. We have collaborated closely together since 1958 when this new method of brachytherapy was initiated at that institution. I am equally grateful to Chahin Chahbazian and to Frank Wilson who undertook the English translation of this book. Their development under Juan del Regato has permitted them to conjugate the French and American schools of radiotherapy. I would like to express my gratitude to my colleagues of the Institut Gustave Roussy who have given me a great deal of critical advice; Andree Dutreix in particular, chief of the Department of Radiation Physics who contributed substantially to every step of my new methodology in dosimetry. I also owe very much to my friends Maurice Tubiana and Jean Dutreix, as well as to the entire technical team of the Department of Curietherapy, in particular Monique Delapierre. I am also indebted to the members of my new team on the service of Radiation Oncology at the Hospital Mondor at Creteil in particular Ginnette Marinello in Radiophysics and Irene Turgard in the technical area. At the Nuclear Center of Saclay, I would like to thank the director of the Department of Radioelements, Charles Fisher, who, with all of his group has succeeded in standardizing the new miniaturized sources of Iridium 192 and Cesium 137. And, lastly, I would like to extend my appreciation to the Centre Antoine-Beclere where I found the invaluable help of their extensive library.

B. PIERQUIN

REFERENCES

1. Pierquin, B., Chassagne, D., and Perz, R.: *Precis deCuriethérapie,* Paris, 1964, Masson et Cie. Edit.
2. I.A.E.A.: *Physical Aspects of Radioisotope Brachytherapy,* technical reports series No. 75, Vienna, 1967.
3. Pierquin B., and Chassagne, D.: La préparation non radioactive en curiethérapie intérstitielle et de contact, *J. de Radiologie, 43:*65-72, 1962.
4. Pierquin, B., and Chassagne, D.: Iridium 192 et le Cesium 137 dans les pérspèctives du récent décret sur la protéction contre les radiations ionisnates, *J. de Radiologie, 49:*533-534, 1968.

CONTENTS

BRACHYTHERAPY

Chapter I

HISTORICAL NOTES

The history of brachytherapy is the story of a French family, the Curies. In a note addressed to the Academie des Sciences on December 26, 1898, Pierre and Marie Curie reported their discovery of a new radioactive substance found in pitchblende, which they named radium. Processing several tons of uranium ore, or pitchblende, they were able to extract a few milligrams of radium chloride in their laboratory at the Municipal School of Physics and Chemistry, rue Vaquelin, on the St. Genevieve Hills. The discovery was made after Becquerel had demonstrated the radioactive properties of uranium in 1896 following the accidental exposure of a photographic plate to uranium crystals in the darkness of a drawer. In 1903, Becquerel and the Curies were awarded the Nobel Prize in Physics.

After the accidental death of Pierre Curie in 1906, Marie Curie pursued her research of radium, determining its atomic weight in 1907 and subsequently succeeding in isolating it in a pure state. In 1911, as a consequence of this later work, she received a second Nobel Prize in Chemistry. Meanwhile, the first tenative therapeutic applications of radium were multiplying throughout the world. In 1901, Danlos and Block irradiated a lesion of lupus at the Hospital St. Louis in Paris. In 1905, Abbe attempted the first interstitial application in the United States, and in the same year Fricke founded the Holt Radium Institute in Manchester. In 1906, Wickham and Degrais created a radium laboratory in Paris with Dominici as clinical director while Danne assumed the production of radium. In 1909, Finze in England succeeded in accomplishing the first application with a 50 milligram tube of radium. However, all of these trials were isolated cases or were performed under unsatisfactory technical conditions. The more proper use of radium was to be discovered later.

At the Pasteur Laboratory of the Institut du Radium of the University of Paris, founded in 1909, Marie Curie pursued her work and studied the clinical applications on which the fundamental techniques of curietherapy were based. Claudius Regaud became director of this institute in 1914, but because of World War I, failed to organize a research team. In 1918, he started to surround himself with laboratory and clinical staff that subsequently made the reputation of the institute. The radiological team initiated by Claudius Regaud and Antoine Lacassagne studied the effects of irradiation on different tissues and established guidelines for the radiotherapy of cancer. With George Richard, Jean Pierquin and Octave Monod as a clinical group, and with the assistance of Henri Coutard in the field of roentgentherapy and Roux-Berger in surgery, the therapeutic rules of optimal dose were gradually established, and the concepts of protraction and fractionation evolved. These developments were realized using "emanation of radium" (radon) which made it possible to easily change the linear activity of the material used. It was with radon that a unit of curietherapy was defined, "the millicure-destroyed" (mcd), a term subsequently abandoned. Following several radionecroses, the concept of filtering the beta radiation and the soft gamma radiation with sheets of gold or platinum was born. In 1923, the "emanation," which was too hazardous to manipulate, was abandoned and was replaced first by the bromate, then by the sulfate of radium, a stable material which was ultimately used in platinum needles and tubes.

Meanwhile, other institutes of radium therapy made their appearance throughout the world; the Radium Hemmett in Stockholm in 1910 under Berg, and the Memorial Hospital of New York in 1913 under Ewing and Janeway, where the exclusive use of lightly filtered radon seeds did not allow a lasting pre-eminence of brachytherapy over sugery. During the 1920's, the Institut du Radium of Paris was expanded on rue d'Ulm with the addition of the Foundation Curie and maintained its leadership of curietherapy, attracting the entire world to pursue the study of radiobiology and radiotherapy. In Paris itself, other centers developed, particularly the Hopital Tenon where Lucien Mallet and Robert Coliez established the foundation of spatial dosimetry utilizing ionization microchambers and developed the concept of isodose curves.

In the 1930's, leadership in brachytherapy moved to Manchester, England, where, at the Holt Radium Institute, Ralston Paterson standardized the rules of radium implantation with dose tables which allowed disengagement from the earlier empiricism, and established the practice of endo-and plesiotherapy based on accurate dosimetry.

In 1934, only 36 years after the discovery of radium, the daughter of Pierre and Marie Curie, Irene Joliet-Curie and her husband Frederic Joliot-Curie, discovered artificial radioactivity. By bombarding a plate of aluminum with alpha rays from a source of polonium, they observed that the aluminum emitted positrons. This emission persisted for a certain time and decreased exponentially after the cessation of the bombardment by alpha particles. They concluded that the bombardment of the aluminum by the alpha particles had produced a new radioactive material, namely, radioactive phosphorus as illustrated by the following reaction:

$$^{27}_{13}\mathrm{A} + {}^{4}_{2}\mathrm{He} \longrightarrow {}^{30}_{15}\mathrm{P} + {}^{1}_{0}\mathrm{n}$$

With this transmutation of matter, artificial radioactivity was born. In 1935, Frederic and Irene Joliot-Curie received the Nobel Prize in Chemistry for this great discovery (3).

The production and therapeutic uses of other radioisotopes had a slow beginning because of limited production capability of cyclotrons. However, at Berkeley, Lawrence made use of the first therapeutic application of radioactive phosphorus in chronic leukemia as early as 1940. Not until after World War II did the development of nuclear reactors make the production of the first sealed sources possible; needles of Cobalt 60 in 1948 by W. G. Myers in the United States, Tantalum 182 pins and gold 198 seeds in 1952 by W. K. Sinclair (5) in England, and Iridium 192 seeds in 1958 by U. K. Henschke in the United States. After having started with gold 198 pins in 1958, we have since standardized and generalized the use of Iridium 192 wires and pins at the Institut Gustave Roussy since 1960, especially in endotherapy. More recently, we have introduced the use of Cesium 137 seeds in gynecological plesiotherapy. All of these new techniques of nonradioactive preparations are controlled by our new dosimetry based on the "Paris System," formerly called Relational System.

REFERENCES

1. Curie, E.: *Madame Curie, Paris,* Paris, 1938, Gallimard Edit.
2. Case, J. T.: The early History of Radiumtherapy and the American Radium Society, *Am. J. of Roentgenology, 82:*574-585, 1959.
3. Strohl, A. Bugnard, M., and Berger, M.: Radio-activité artificielle, in Delherm, L.: Eléctroradiothérapie, 1:685-730, Paris, 1951, Masson et Cie, Edit.
4. Myers. W. G.: Application of artificial radioactive isotopes in therapy; Cobalt 60. *Am. J. of Roentgenology, 60:*816-823, 1948.
5. Sinclair, W. K.: Artificial radioactive sources for interstitial Therapy, *Brit. J. of Radiology, 25:*417-419, 1952.
6. Pierquin, B.: Endo et plésio-radiothérapie par Iridium 192 et Cesium 137, *Radiol. Clin. Biol., 35:*407-418, 1966.

Chapter II

PHYSICAL NOTES

These notes will be brief since this book is not meant to dwell extensively on the details of physics of radiations which are available at length in excellent works under the authorship of M. Tubiana, A. and J. Dutreix (1). We will be satisfied to review some definitions of physical terms currently used in radiotherapy and in particular in brachytherapy.

Isotopes are atoms of different atomic masses but the same atomic number Z (Z = number of protons), therefore, the same nuclear charges with the same number of peripheral electrons and the same chemical properties.

In conventional nuclear notion, the letter Z at the lower left of the chemical symbol is the atomic number and represents the number of protons in the nucleus of the atom. The letter A at the upper left of the chemical symbol is the *mass number:* A = Z protons + N neutrons. For example:

$$^{A}_{Z}X$$

when the chemical nature of an element is specified, there is no possible error as to its atomic number and often only its mass number is mentioned; for example, $^{32}_{15}P$ is currently referred to as P -32.

The radioactivity of an atom is the result of a violent reaction between the nucleons, called disintegration, with the ejection of particles from the nucleus and often associated with the production of a certain quantity of energy in the form of photons.

Electron capture, commonly called "K capture," is a consequence of a particular transmutation of the radioactive nucleus which incorporates an electron from the K shell, or less commonly from the L shell, with transformation of a proton into a neutron within the nucleus. The ionization produced at the K shell by the loss of an electron provokes a cascade of more peripheral electrons with the emission of fluorescent photons. The relatively low energies of these fluorescent photons, which are x rays because of their extranuclear origin, are of particular interest in endo- and plesiotherapy. The problem of protection would be considerably simplified if they could be used routinely.

Beta radiation is corpuscular radiation emitted as a continuous spectrum of energies varying between 0 and a maximal value according to a distribution which is particular and characteristic for each radio-emitter. The beta rays are electrons mostly of negative charge (negatrons), occasionally with a positive charge (positrons) and symbolized by the Greek letter β.

Gamma radiation is electromagnetic radiation emitted in the form of a discontinuous spectrum with gamma rays of different energies which are characteristic for each radioactive element. Gamma rays are photons symbolized by the Greek letter γ.

The *nuclear reactor* for atomic piles consists of equipment in which the controlled fission of Uranium 235 produces a continuous and constant flux of neutrons. In atomic piles, this flux reaches and exceeds 10^{12} neutrons/cm ^{2}/sec. A sample that is placed in this flux for activation will be transformed into radioactive isotopes by the introduction of neutrons into its nuclei. In most instances, this process will bring about either a neutron-gamma reaction (n), or a neutron-proton reaction **(n,p)** The neutron-gamma reaction is by far the most frequent. It is illustrated as follows:

$$^{A-1}X(n, \gamma)^{A}X$$

One can also use fission byproducts such as Cesium 137.

The *cyclotron* and the *synchrocyclotron* will accelerate positive ions in circular trajectories under the influences of a perpendicualr magnetic field. In most instances, at the level of the irradiated sample, deuterons (^2_1H) yield nuclear reactions of different types: deuteron-neutron (d,n), deuteron-alpha (d,α) and especially deuteron-proton (d,p).

The unit of radioactivity - The Curie. Its initial definition was that quantity of radon in radioactive equilibrium with 1 gram of radium. The decay of 1 gram of radium is at the rate of 3.7 x 10^{10} disintegrations/second. We have maintained this unit of radioactivity for all artificially radioactive elements.

The curie is, therefore, that quantity of any radioactive element that decays at the rate of 3.7×10^{10} disintegrations/second. In practice, we use only small fractions of this unit in endo- and plesiotherapy: usually 1,000th of a curie, the millicurie or quantity of radioactive element that decays at the rate of 3.7 x 10 disintegrations/second.

The symbol for millicurie is mCi. A new unit, the Becquerel, has recently been adopted by the ICRU.

The *mass activity* is the radioactivity of 1 gram of a substance or the number of disintegrations per unit of time in 1 gram of this substance. In practice, the specific activity is measured in millicuries per gram (mCi/g.).

The *cross section* applies to a sample irradiated in a flux of neutrons, and is an index of the probability with which neutrons will be stopped by the atomic nuclei of the irradiated substance. The unit of cross section is the "barn." The greater the cross section of the substance, the higher its specific activity.

The *half life* is the time in which the initial number of radioactive atoms is reduced by one half. The decay of radioactive elements follows an exponential curve in relation to time; it is, therefore, represented by a straight line on a semi-logarithmic scale symbolized by the letter $T^{1/2}$ (Figure 1).

The *average life* is equal to the total duration of individual lives of all radioactive atoms present divided by their number. It is as if the initial number of disintegrations were constant for the entire duration of this average life. It is symbolized by the Greek letter $\theta = 1.44T^{1/2}$. The average life is very useful when one wishes to study the total number of disintegrations (for example: the total dose delivered by a radioactive element left permanently in a tumor) (Figure 2).

The *exposure rate constant,* currently called Γ factor represents the exposure rate per unit of time at a distance of 1 cm from a point source of 1 mCi. It is symbolized by the letter Γ and is expressed in $R/mCi/h/cm^2$.

The classical unit of *linear activity* is mCi/cm and is used throughout this text. However, a new specification has been recently suggested by A. Dutreix and is recommended by the N. C. R. P. This unit, the *linear nominal output* is expressed in milliroentgens hour/centimeter of active length at 1 meter.

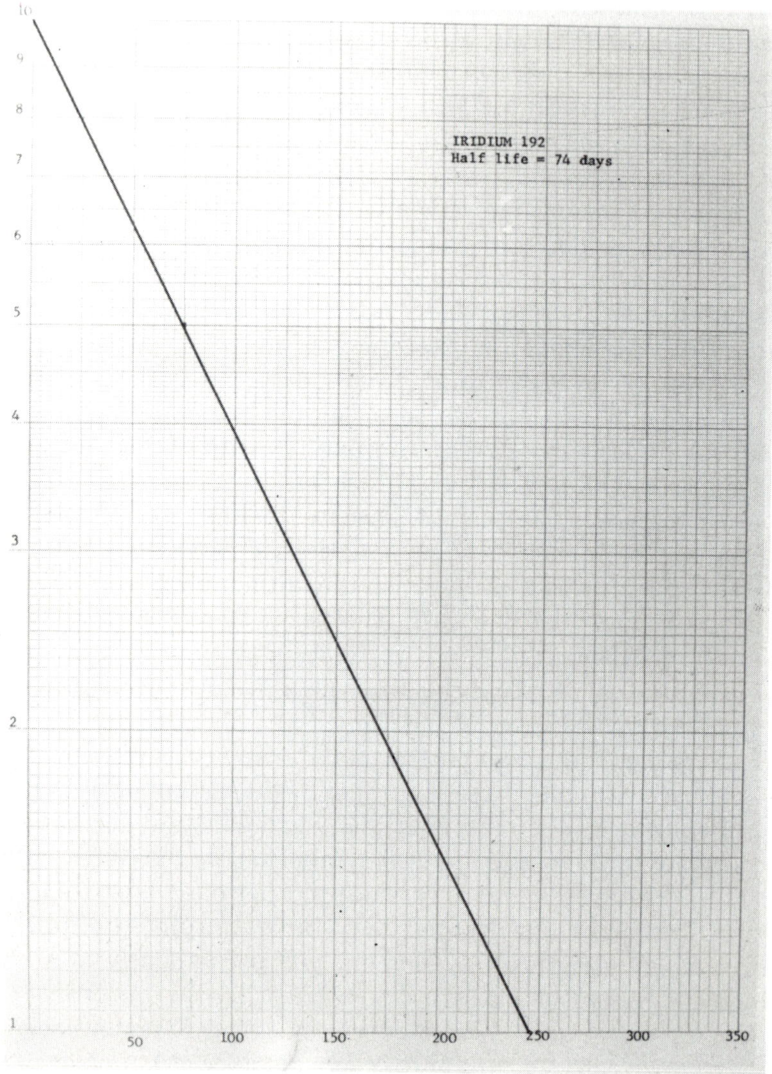

Figure 1. The radioactive decay of Iridium 192. (semi logarithmic coordinates)

The *half value layer* commonly abbreviated by the initials HVL is the thickness of a defined material required to attenuate half the incident radiations. The HVL is usually expressed in lead; a material commonly used for protection.

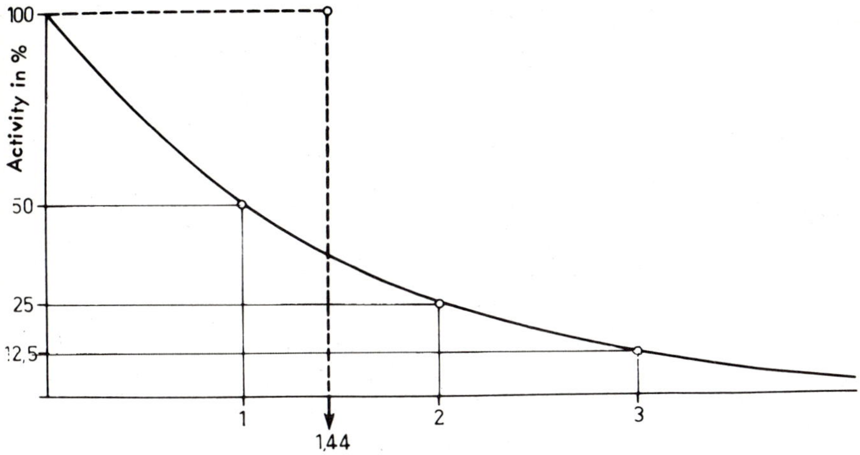

Figure 2. Graphic representation of half life and average life
_________exponential decay curve
- - - - - - - - average life (θ=1.44)

REFERENCES

1. Tubiana, M., Dutreix, J., Dutreix, A., and Jockey, P.: *Bases Physiques de la radiobiologie,* Paris, 1963, Masson et Cie Edit.
2. *Specification of Gamma Ray Brachytherapy Sources,* Report 41, Washington, D. C., NCRP, 1974.

Chapter III

THE RADIOACTIVE MATERIALS

As we indicated in our introduction, we foresee the use of sealed radioactive sources only, which are safer to use and free of the risk of contaminating the facilities, the personnel and the patients. They include:

1) Phosphorus 32

Half life: 14.3 days

Maximum energy of its beta particles: 1.7 MeV.

As a pure beta emitter, phosphorus 32 is indicated in the plesiotherapy of the skin. Incorporated in vinyl chloride, it is used as an applicator in the form of discs 70 mm in diameter composed of an active layer 1 mm thick and an inactive layer 2 mm thick. The active surface is red in color; the inactive surface is colorless. They can easily be shaped by cutting them with scissors. The output at their surface is of the order of 1,500 R/hr. (1)

2) Strontium 90

Half life: 28 years

Maximum energy of its beta particles: 0.5 MeV.

It decays to Yttrium 90 which yields beta particles of much higher energies.

As a pure beta emitter, Strontium 90 is used in plesiotherapy of the skin. Totally sealed in a metallic plaque, it is used as a rigid applicator either in the form of a disc 15 mm in diameter or as square applicators of various sizes (Amersham). The active element is Yttrium 90.

The output at the surface of the applicators is approximately 50 to 1200 R/min. (1)

3) Yttrium 90

Half life: 2.7 days.

Maximum energy of its beta particles: 2.26 MeV.

As a pure beta emitter, Yttrium 90 is used in endotherapy. As Yttrium oxide, it can be used either directly in seeds 1.3 mm in diameter and 5 mm in length, especially in pituitary implantations, or in seeds 0.6 mm in diameter and 5 mm in length encased in stainless steel needles with walls 0.1 mm thick and 1 mm. in external diameter as for hemangiomas. Their activity varies between 1 and 2 mCi per seed (2).

4) Cesium 137

Half life: 29.4 years

Average life of its gamma rays: 0.66 MeV.

HVL: 4 mm of lead

Γ factor: 3.3

As a gamma emitter, Cesium 137 is used in endotherapy of small volume implants, especially in gynecological plesiotherapy. A product of fission, it is incorporated in nonpliable ceramic (pollucite) which is resistant to high temperatures with a melting point of 1700°C.

In endotherapy, it consists of a pollucite wire 0.24 mm in diameter introduced into a steel needle with a wall thickness of 0.35 mm and an external diameter of 1.65 mm (Figure 4).

For plesiotherapy, pollucite seeds 0.8 mm thick are sealed within a small steel ball. This sealed seed of Cesium 137 has an external diameter of 1.5 mm and a length of 3.5 mm (Figure 3 (a)) with an activity of the order of 15 mCi. These seeds can be assembled as a chain of sources with inactive interspaces or in steel tubes similar to radium tubes (Figure 3 (b)) (3).

5) Iridium 192

Half life: 74 days

Average energy of its gamma rays: 0.31 MeV.

HVL: 2 mm of lead.

Γ factor: 4.8

As a gamma emitter, Iridium 192 is fundamentally indicated in the endotherapy of all volumes and in some cases of plesiotherapy of the upper airway passages and in the pelvis.

It is in the form of wires composed of an alloy of 25% Iridium, 75% platinum enveloped in pure platinum. This layer of pure platinum absorbs most of the beta radiation. Two sizes are available:

a) A small 0.1 mm in diameter wire of iridized platinum enveloped in pure platinum 0.1 mm thick, therefore, with a total external diameter of 0.3 mm.

b) A large diameter wire of 0.3 mm of iridized platinum enveloped

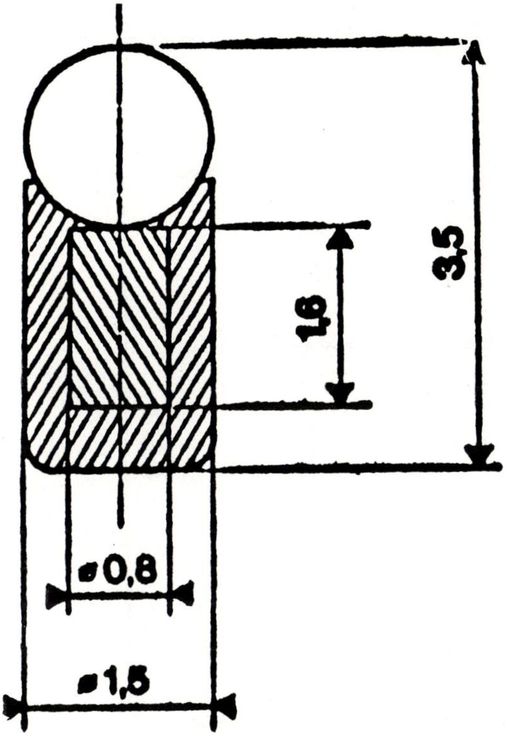

Figure 3a. Diagram of a single cesium 137 seed in its steel envelope.

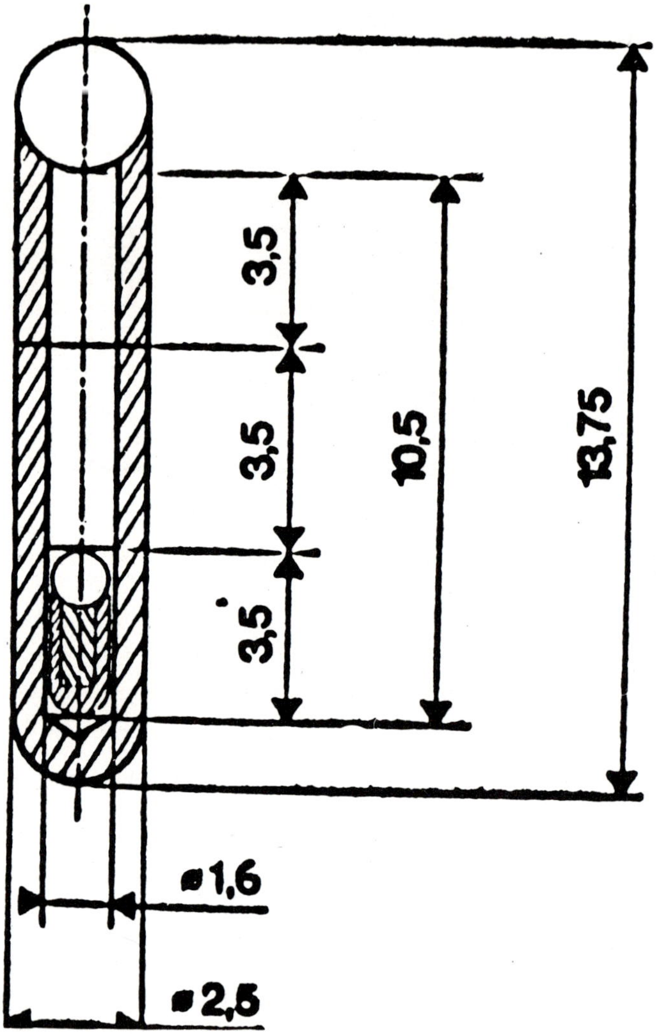

Figure 3b. Diagram of a cesium 137 tube containing 3 cesium seeds. Wall thickness of 0.5 mm.

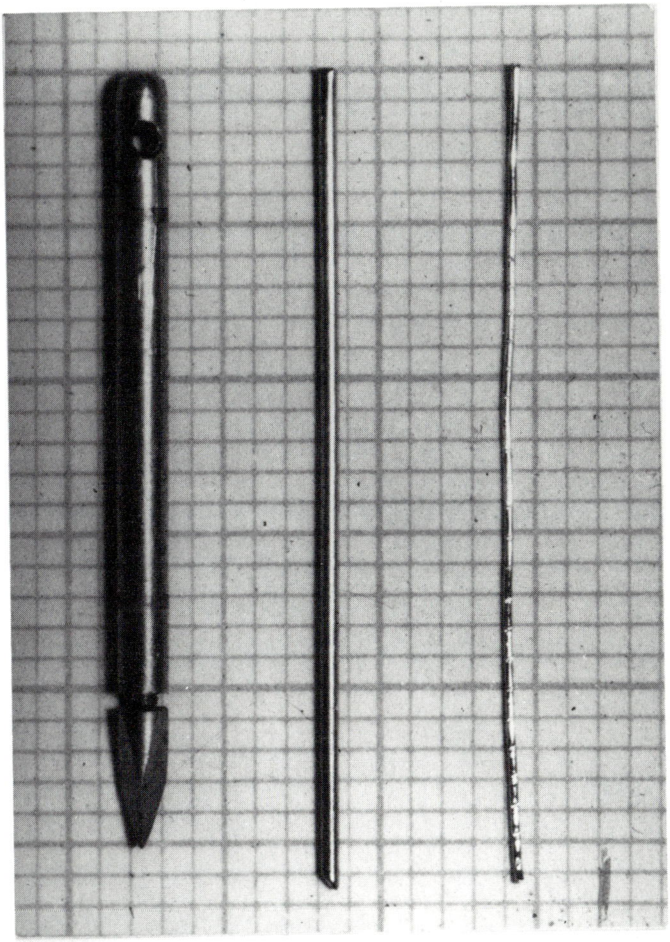

Figure 4. Comparison of a cesium needle 1.7 mm in diameter, an 1^{192} wire 0.5 mm in diameter and a 1^{192} wire 0.3 mm in diameter.

in pure platinum 0.1 mm thick, therefore, with an external diameter of 0.5 mm (Figure 4).

The smaller diameter wire is loaded either into plastic tubes, hypodermic needles or silk sutures, while the larger diameter wire is implanted using guide gutters.

These wires are extremely resistant and nonbreakable, yet highly malleable. The unusually high cross section of Iridium 192 (360 barns) yields a very high specific activity. In endotherapy the linear activity varies between 0.5 and 2.5 mCi/cm. For plesiotherapy, the linear activity varies between 5 and 10 mCi/cm.

Although Iridium wires are not a true sealed source, they are internationally accepted as sealed sources by radiation protection agencies since they do not contaminate cutting instruments and do not release active particles.

REFERENCES

1. Pierquin, B.: La bétathérapie des angiomes par les radio-éléments artificiels, *Annales de Chirugie Plastique, 9:*285-289, 1964.
2. Pierquin, B., Mortreuil, M., Beyer, H., Chassagne, D., and Galle, P.: Les aiguilles d'Yttrium 90 en endo-éléctron — Curiétherapie, *Jour de Radiologie, 45:*78-81. 1964.
3. Pierquin, B: "L'emploi du Cesium 137 en gynécologie," *Annales de Radiol, 10:*11-12, 1962.
4. Pierquin, B.: Endo et plésioradiothérapie par l'Iridium 192 et Cesium 137, *Radiol. Clin. Biol., 35:*407-418, 1966.

Chapter IV

THE TECHNIQUES

At the outset, we must insist on the fundamental importance of afterloading techniques to protect the operator and his assistants. Radiation exposure of the medical personnel when using radium was, in fact, the major obstacle to the full development of curietherapy. The problem of protection is today even more important due to international regulations minimizing the maximum permissible dose for occupationally exposed persons.

The two established protection factors are distance and time. The distance factor should not be neglected since it is of great importance in the organization of a department of brachytherapy, particularly in storing radioactive sources. During a radioactive application, one can "condense" distance with screens of high density material such as lead, for at least part of the personnel. However, at the time of surgery, the radiotherapist should be free from any interposed obstacles and add the screens later. Time is a protection factor used to advantage during the implantation of the radioactive sources. To gain time, one operates quickly; although the correct placement of radioactive sources cannot be accomplished in a rush. As in all forms of modern surgery, technical progress in brachytherapy cannot be assured except by working meticulously, thus prolonging the application time. For these reasons, afterloading techniques had to be developed.

Any progress in brachytherapy depends upon the meticulous applications of radioactive sources in a tumor volume using an adequate sense of sight and, especially, an adequate sense of touch. In fact, it is by palpation that one can most precisely determine the relative position of each radioactive source in relation to the boundaries of the tumor. It is also by palpation that one can modify the treated volume, patiently correcting the position of the sources to finally obtain an evenly spaced setup uniformly covering the entire tumor.

It is evident that a satisfactory application of sources cannot be obtained without using nonradioactive guides prior to placing the radioactive materials so that the operating finger can follow closely and without risk.

The entire nonradioactive application is then controlled radiographically. As much of the dosimetric control (standard roentgenograms, tomograms) as possible should also be secured during the nonradioactive phase.

We will describe only the five main techniques of photon brachytherapy. The techniques with electrons, the indications of which are very limited, are described in appropriate chapters.

1) Guide Gutter Technique (Iridium 192)

(Technique of Pierquin and Chassagne)

General indications — Endotherapy
all anatomic sites
small or average target volumes

Two standard pins of wire 0.5 mm in diameter available.(1)

The hairpin consists of two parallel branches varying in length from 20 to 50 mm each. In routine use, the branches are 40 mm in length and can be shorter if necessary, depending on the requirements of the target volume. They are separated by 12 mm and joined at their head by a transverse branch indented at its center to resemble the shape of the letter "M" to prevent sutures from sliding over the parallel branches. It is shaped prior to being activated by molding the head and by separating its branches slightly.

The single pin is a simple wire, one end of which is tied around itself so that an eyelet is made through which a silk suture can be passed.

The pins are shaped at the Nuclear Center of Saclay before they are irradiated with neutrons for about 30 hours under a flux of 2.6×10^{12}cm^2/sec. yielding, at the time of their therapeutic use, an activity of 0.5 to 2.5mCi/cm.

These pins cannot be directly placed into tissue because they are not sufficiently rigid. It is indispensable that they be implanted using rigid guide materials offering a second essential advantage, that of planning the implantation with a nonradioactive material. The operator can, therefore, in complete safety and with detailed radiographic control, possibly followed by corrections, execute the actual application. The guide materials are either twin or single

guide gutters made of stainless steel, a description of which follows:
a) Twin Guide Gutters or Slotted Hairpin Guides (Figure 5)

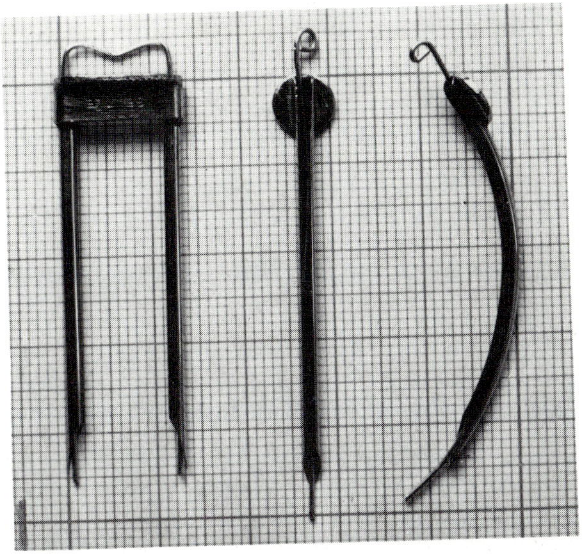

Figure 5. Double and single guide gutters containing 1^{192} hairpin and single pins.

The parallel tubes of the guide gutters have an external diameter of 1.8 mm with an internal diameter of 1.4 mm. A 0.7 mm wide longitudinal aperture allows the radioactive wire to enter the tubes with a margin of 0.2 mm. A slightly funneled aperture at the entrance of the tube facilitates the introduction of the branches of the pin and the transit of its head. The two parallel tubes are separated from each other by a distance of 12 mm and are joined at their superior end by a small metallic plaque 5 mm in height with a small lip on its external side allowing a solid grip during the instrumentation, a technical detail that is essential. The longitudinal apertures of the tubes are located medially, and facing each other to prevent the wires, the elasticity of which tends to separate the two branches of the pin, from slipping out during the insertion of the radioactive sources. Twin guide gutters are made in lengths of 30, 40 and 50 mm.

b) Single Guide Gutters or Slotted Guide Needles

Two types of single guides are available:

1. Straight guides with lengths varying between 30 and 70 mm.
2. Curved guides with a radius of 35 mm and a length of 40 mm.

The heads of these tubes lie on a small metallic plaque 10 mm in diameter to permit holding it with forceps. Their aperture is on the side opposite the small metallic plaque, and on the concave side of curved guides (Figure 5).

The application of the pin is carried out in the following manner: first the cannular guides are implanted in the tumor under local or general anesthesia. With the help of fluoroscopy, one verifies their exact position and corrects any misplacement. With a curved needle, nylon sutures are placed in position by passing them under the head of the twin guides in a plane perpendicular to the transverse plaque and equidistant from the two branches. For single guides, the nylon suture is placed around the head in the same manner as around the head of a radium needle. The ends of each suture are left untied, marked and held with hemostats. The radioactive pins are then taken from lead containers and rapidly inserted into the guide gutters as follows:

The operator verifies the parallelism of the two branches of the pin with the help of two nonserrated forceps with flat tips by applying slight torion of a few degrees externally at the end of each branch(Figure6(a)).

With the help of the nonserrated forceps in one hand, he then grasps the midportion of one of the vertical branches of the hairpin at an angle so that its two branches are introduced in the same axis as that of the guide gutter.

With another nonserrated forceps in the other hand, the lip of the guide is gripped holding it tightly.

The loose branch of the pin is first introduced into the corresponding tube for a length of 3 to 6 mm.

The branch held with the forceps is then introduced into the second tube by rotating it slightly clockwise around the head of the guide (Figure 6 (b)).

The operator then releases the hairpin which should remain in place at the entrance of the tubes from the mere expansibility of its branches and the slight separation of its ends. He will, however,

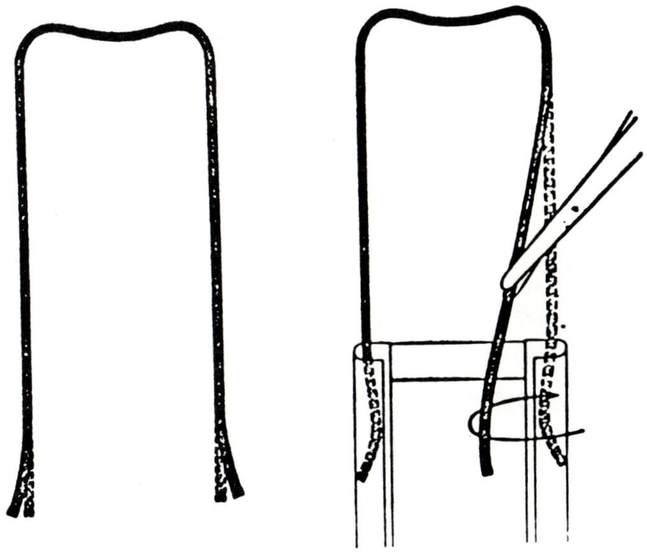

Figure 6a. Slight spreading of tips of I^{192} hairpin prior to insertion.

Figure 6b. Technique of introducing hairpin into guide gutter.

continue holding the twin guide firmly with the other forceps.

The hairpin is then inserted through the total length of the twin guide by simply tapping lightly on the head at the central depression in the transverse branch with the free forceps in a closed position, used as a small hammer. The pin should slide easily all along the length of the tubes without meeting resistance. If any resistance is encountered in this process, we recommend against forcing the pin. It is probably due to escape of one of the branches of the pin from the guide gutter. When this occurs, the pin should be removed, reshaped and reintroduced in the usual way.

Once the pin reaches the neck of the twin cannular guide, the latter is removed from the tissues leaving the pin in place. In order to retain the pin in place during this process, a surgical hook is placed on the transverse branch of the pin at the level of the central depression. The operator can then extract the twin guide by pulling it gently and carefully by its lip to facilitate the sliding of the pin against the metallic plaque of the guide.

As soon as the transverse branch of the pin appears under the transverse plaque of the twin guide, the operator holds it tightly in place and the guide gutter can then be rapidly extracted with a quick movement of the other hand (Figure 6 (c)).

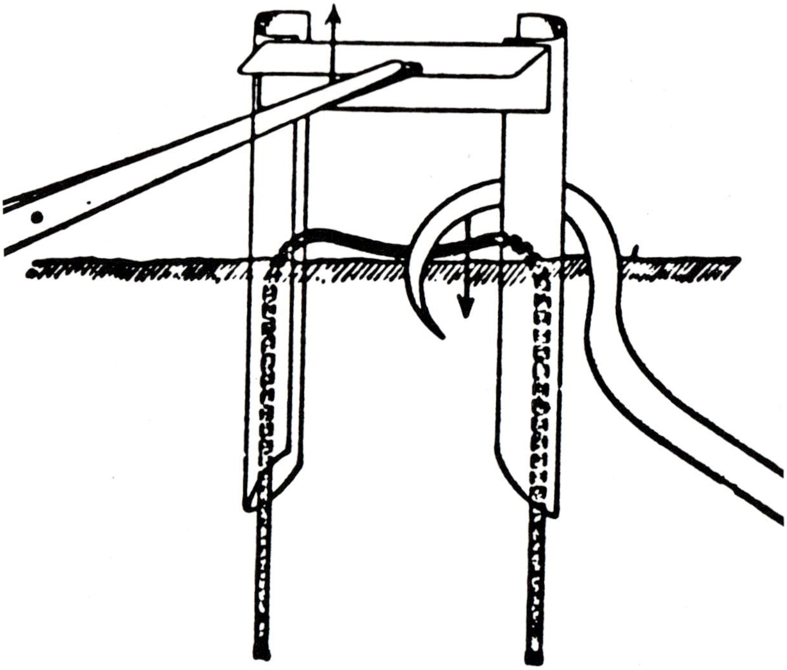

Figure 6c. Technique of substituting hairpin for the guide gutter. The surgical hook maintains the head of the pin in contact with the mucosa.

In expert hands, the entire procedure of inserting and substituting a hairpin can be performed very rapidly in about 15 to 30 seconds.

In the case of curved single guides, the wire should be given a corresponding curvature by molding it with the forceps beforehand. After pushing the pin through the length of the tubes, the latter are removed from the tissues while the operator simultaneously maintains each pin in place. Only the head of the pin projects slightly above the surface of the implanted area.

Nylon sutures are tied over the hairpin at the level of its central depression. In the case of simple pins, one end of the nylon suture is threaded through the eye, being careful to maintain the pin in place with the help of forceps while the knot is secured. Threading the eye of the simple pin can be facilitated by using a seamstresses needle threader (Figure 7 (a, b, c)).

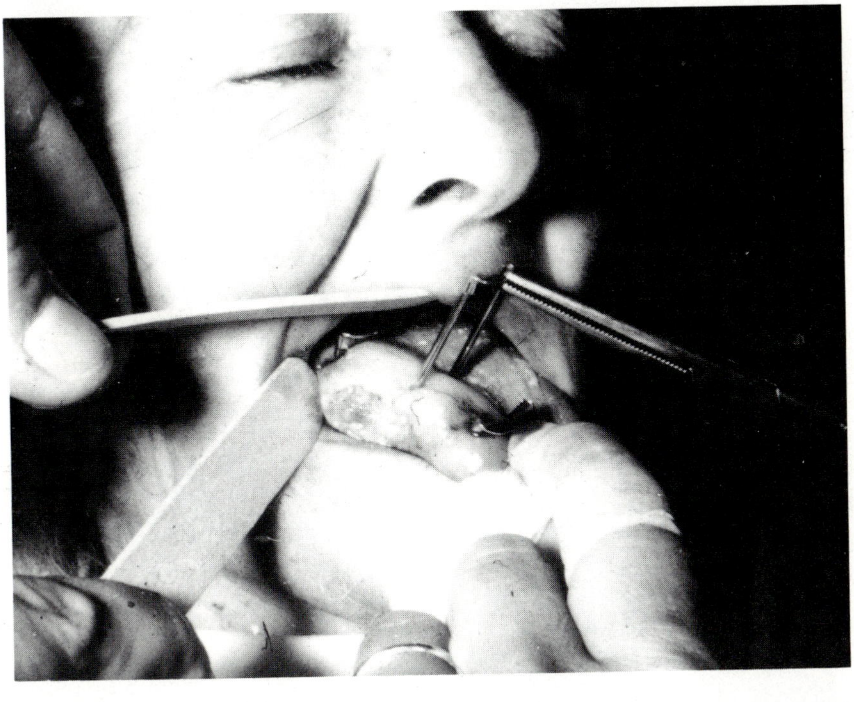

Figure 7a. Cancer of the mobile tongue. Implantation of 3 double guide gutters.

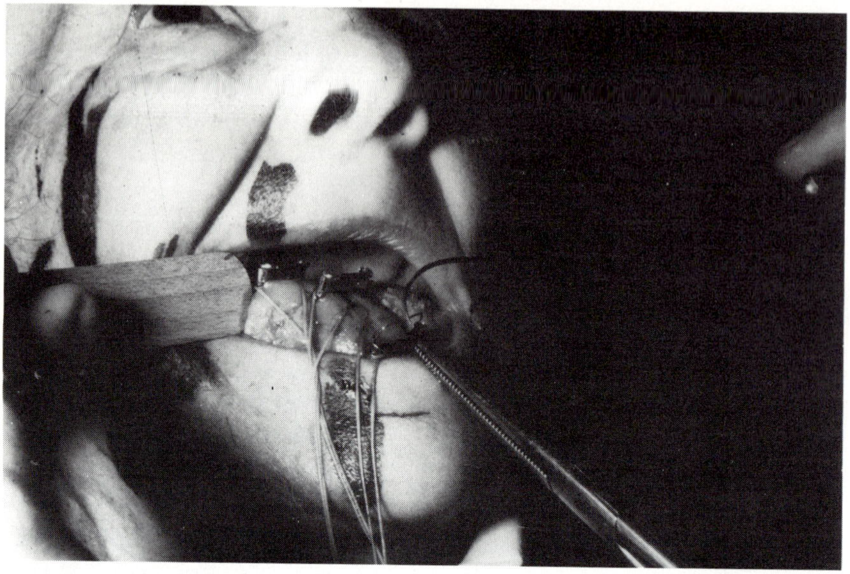

Figure 7b. Cancer of the mobile tongue. Insertion of radioactive hairpins into implanted guides gutters. Skin marks for later tomography.

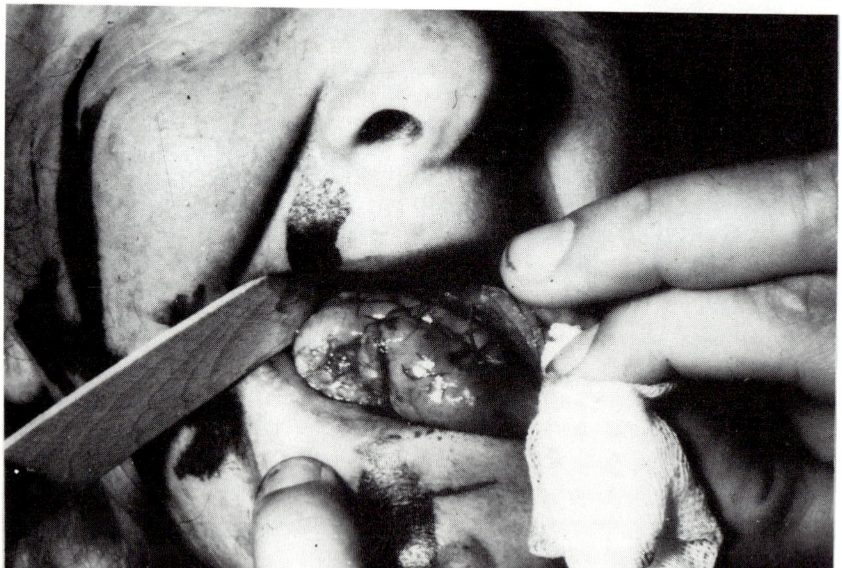

Figure 7c. Cancer of the mobile tongue. I^{192} hairpins have been substituted for each guide gutter and sutured to the mucosa.

In these maneuvers, it is essential to use pin-carrying forceps with nonserrated, slightly flat ends. The operator should hold the materials gently and be able to work delicately without locking pin-carrying or tube-carrying forceps.

2) Plastic Tube Technique (Henschke's Technique)

General Indications
Endotherapy
Plesiotherapy
All anatomic sites
Average and large target volumes

This technique transfixes skin and requires leaving a permanent guide material in place during the entire duration of the application. This is accomplished using plastic tubes into which Iridium 192 wires are afterloaded. This technique was fundamentally perfected by Henschke. We have modified it very slightly(2).

The radioactive wire, 0.3 mm in diameter, is inserted into plastic tubing with an internal diameter of 0.5 mm and an external diameter of 0.85 mm. This small "inner" tube is cut to a convenient length and then from behind a lead screen using two long forceps, the operator eases the Iridium wires into one end of these plastic tubes with successive small pushes until the end of the wire is flush with the end of the tube. The slight natural curvature of the wire is usually sufficient to maintain it well in place within the tube. The other end of the tube is labeled with adhesive tape indicating the number, the delivery date and the length of the Iridium wire. The radioactive segment of this Iridium 192 wire carrier is placed in a multichannel container with a capacity for about 20 tubes and is ready to be transported to the operating room (Figure 8 (a, b)). A modification of this technique was recently proposed by A. Sahatchiev and M. Mouchmov using silk sutures to carry the Iridium 192 wires.

The "outer" guide system for these "inner" tubes is composed of the following (Figure 9):

1. Stainless steel needles with an internal diameter of 1.2 mm and an external diameter of 1.6 mm in standard lengths of 15, 20 and 30 cm.
2. "Outer" large plastic tubes of similar diameter.

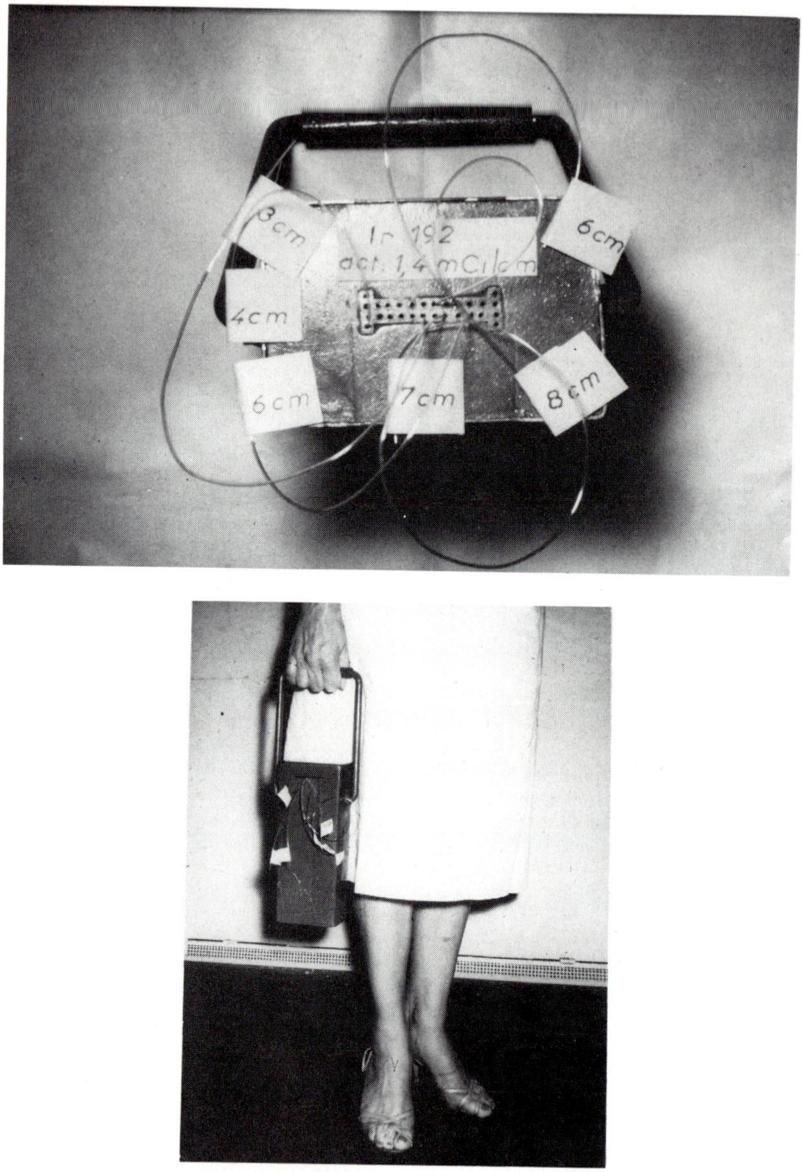

Figure 8. The portable container for plastic tubes loaded with I^{192} wires. Wall thickness = 3 cm. lead minimum.

a. Top view showing multichannel capacity.

b. Side view showing lateral window in the container cover for the exit of the tubes.

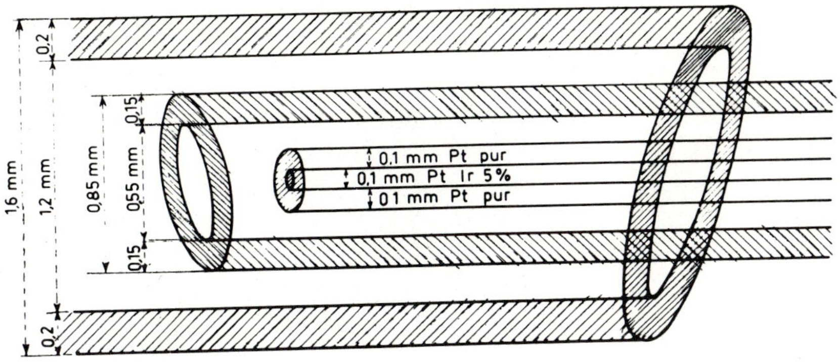

Figure 9. Plastic tube technique
Diagram of 1^{192} wire, small "inner" plastic tube, and large "outer" plastic tube.

3. Stainless steel obturators 1 mm in diameter, 25 cm long or nylon thread 0.8 to 0.9 mm in diameter.

4. Metallic immobilization buttons with a nippled central hole 3 mm long and 1.7 mm in diameter that can be threaded onto the ends of either the stainless steel needle or the outer plastic tubes.

Their application in the target volume is performed in the following manner:

The guide needles are implanted in the target volume transcutaneously and successively in one or several planes making their exit through the skin at the opposite side of the target volume. Their spacing and parallelism can be verified with the help of fluoroscopy and by directly viewing their ends which remain free in the air at their entrance and exit (Figure 10).

For each guide needle, the substitution of outer plastic tubes is performed in one of two ways:

A) Pushing Method of Substitution

a) With the aid of an obturator inside the guide needle, the outer plastic tube is slid over the tip of the needle. A sufficient length of the obturator is left inside the plastic tube to enable carrying the plastic tube through the entire length of the implanted volume. Pushing the coupled obturator and plastic tube with one hand, the operator guides the exit of the needle with the other and substitutes the large plastic tube for the guide needle which is removed from the tissues together with the obturator. When the plastic tube reaches the exit,

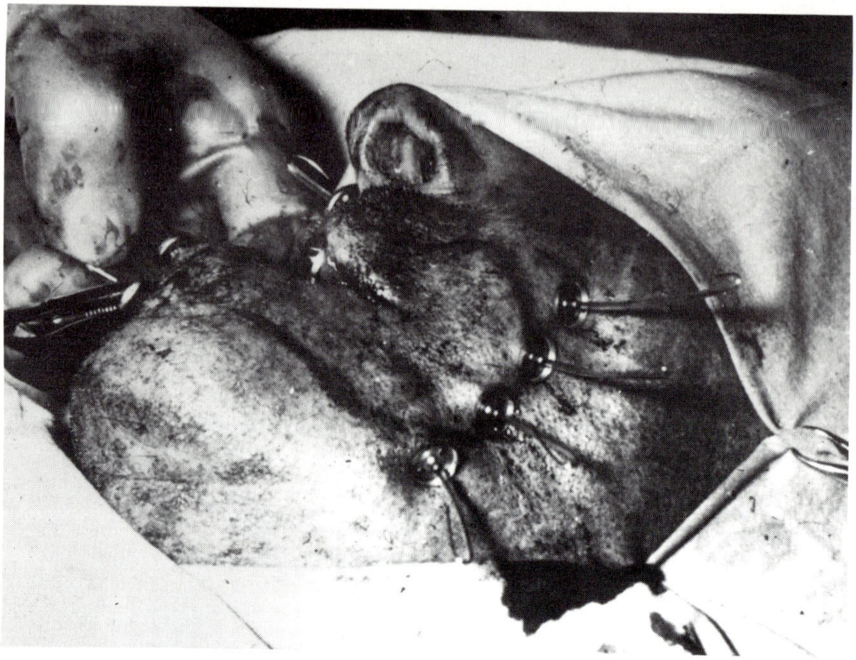

Figure 10. Plastic tube technique. Cancer of the buccal mucosa. 4 plastic tubes containing dummy sources for dosimetry. Immobilization buttons in position.

one has to push it more forcefully in order to push it through the skin. This is facilitated by simultaneously exerting counterpressure on the surface of the skin with the thumb and index finger. The outer plastic tubes are thus successively placed in position allowing 4 to 5 cm of tube to protrude beyond the skin at either end.

b) Metallic immobilization buttons are slid over the ends of the individual tubes and brought in contact with the skin.

c. A dilute solution of heparin is injected into each tube in order to avoid clotting of blood within the tubes prior to the loading of the radioactive sources.

d. Lead wires with lengths equal to planned radioactive sources for each tube are then introduced into the plastic tubes as dummy sources for marker films and tomography.

e) The dosimetry is completed and the last corrections are made.

f) The inner plastic tubes carrying the Iridium 192 are inserted into the outer plastic tubes, after the removal of the inactive wires. Using long forceps to gently hold the outer tube, the inner tubes are pushed into their correct position.

g) The inner tubes are immobilized by crushing the nipple of the immobilization buttons to fix the two tubes together.

B) Pulling Method of Substitution (Raynal's Technique). In this method, the metallic obturator is replaced by solid nylon thread. This thread is sold commercially as "fishing thread." Its flexibility and strength make it an ideal material for forming loops around tumors situated in natural cavities where instrumentation is difficult. To illustrate this very simple and efficient technical modification, the technique of making a loop for treating an infiltrating carcinoma of the base of the tongue is illustrated in (Figures 11 a through l). This modification facilitates the use of plastic tubes whenever such loops are necessary.

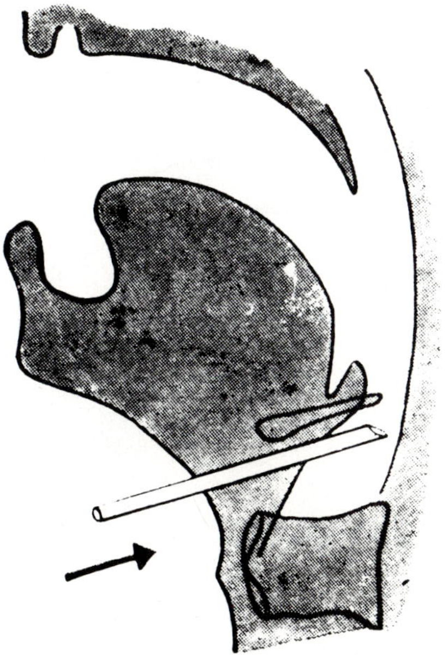

Figure 11. Base of Tongue. Formation of a loop. Plastic tube Technique of Raynal.

a. Implantation of 1st guide needle.

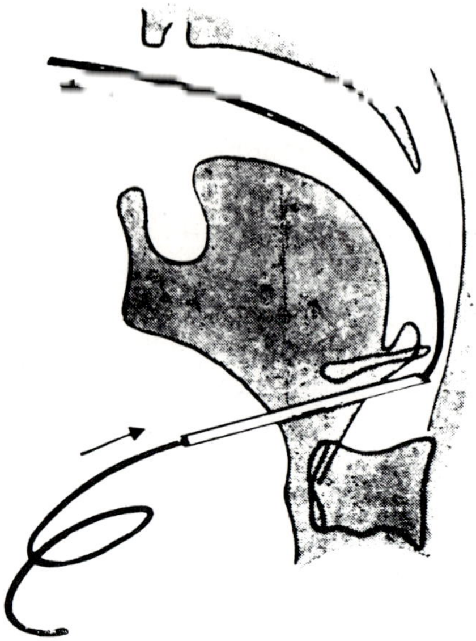

Figure 11. b. a 40 cm long nylon cord is passed through guide needle exiting through mouth

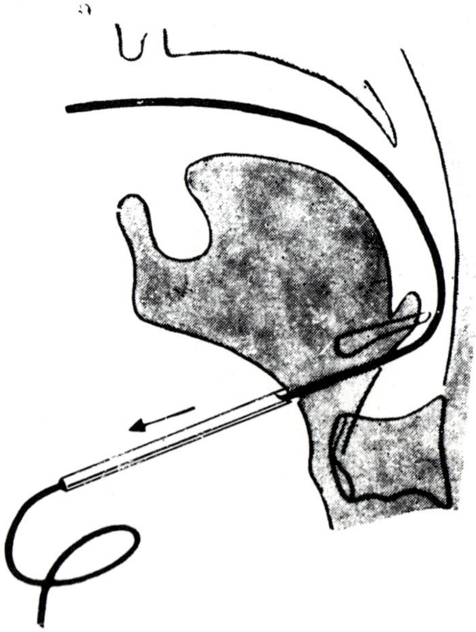

Figure 11. c. extraction of guide needle

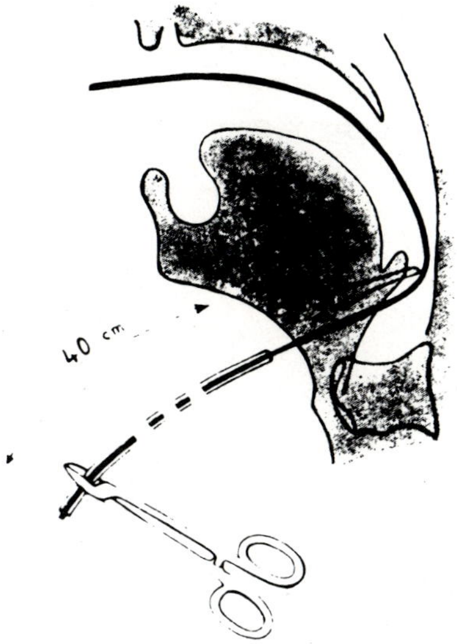

Figure 11.
d. Plastic tube is fixed to nylopn cord with small clamp.

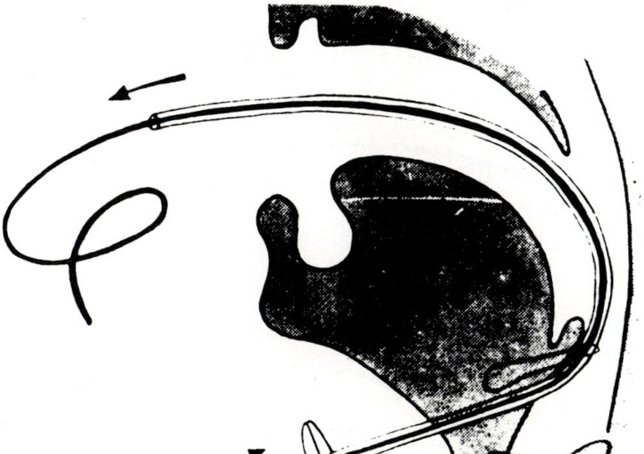

Figure 11.
e. Using firm quick tug plastic tube traverses skin, muscle and muscosa replacing nylon cord which is removed.

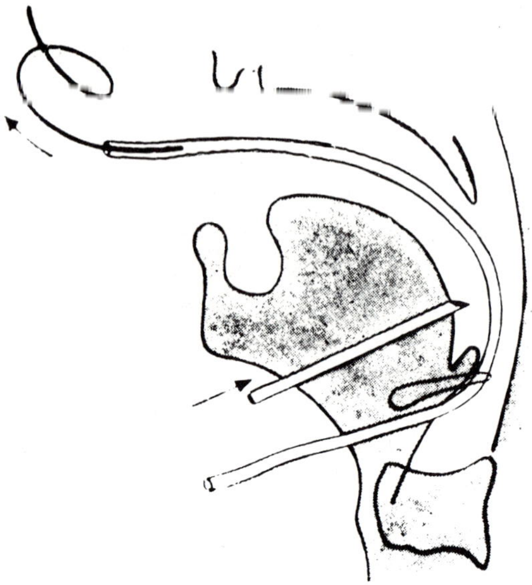

Figure 11.
f. Implantation of 2nd needle.

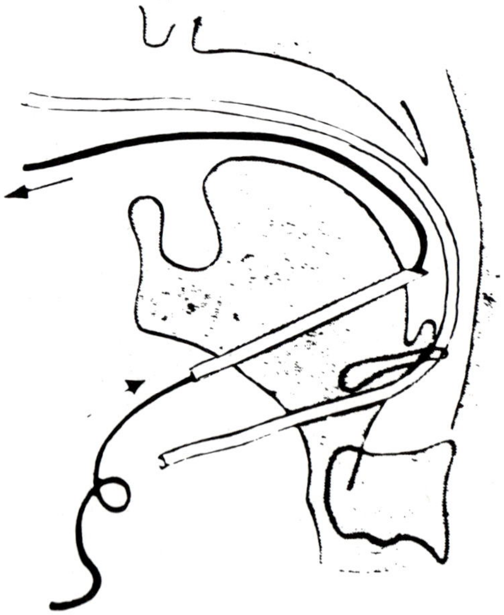

Figure 11.
g. Reinsertion of nylon cord.

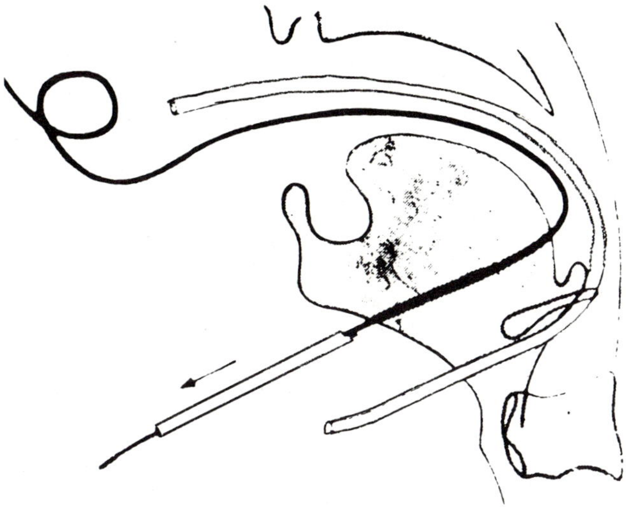

Figure 11.
h. Extraction of 2nd needle.

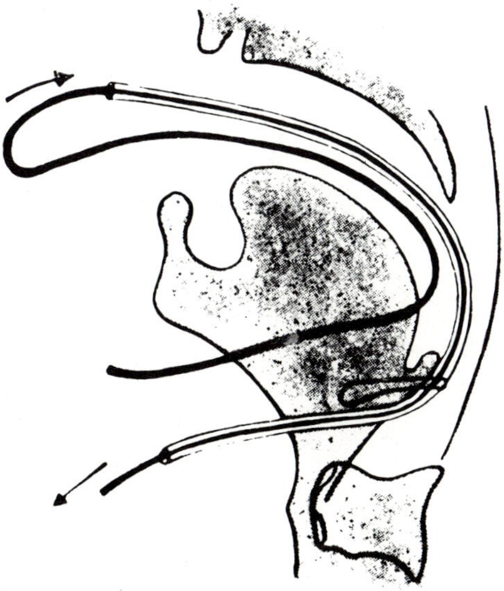

Figure 11.
i. The nylon cord is passed completely through the plasic tube.

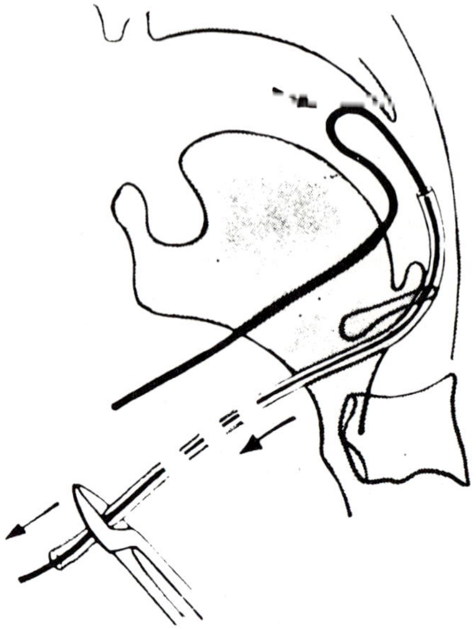

Figure 11.
j. Tip of plastic tube is brought into contact with base of tongue.

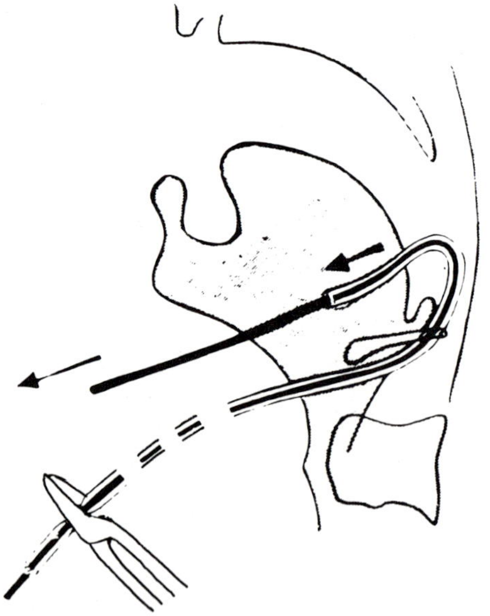

Figure 11.
k. By pulling nylon cord and with digital pressure on the tube in the oropharynx it is pulled through mueosa, muscles and skin.

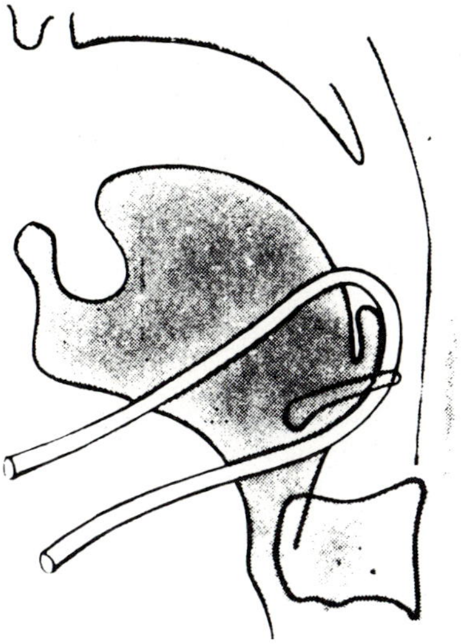

Figure 11.
1. Following removal of nylon cord and clamp the completed loop is ready for afterloading.

3) Hypodermic Needle Technique (Pierquin's Technique)

General Indications:

Endotherapy

Skin or accessible mucous membranes.

Small or average target volumes

This method uses a transfixation technique in which the guide materials are nickle hypodermic needles beveled at both ends and having an external diameter of 0.8 mm and an internal diameter of 0.5 mm. Their length varies between 2 and 8 cm in 1 cm intervals.

The Iridium 192 wire, 0.3 mm in diameter, is introduced in the same manner as an obturator (Figure 12 (a)).

After establishing the target volume, hypodermic needles of appropriate lengths are chosen, remembering to select needles which are longer than the tumor volume to allow a sufficient margin of irradiation. For a tumor 2 cm in diameter, a needle approximately 4 cm long as needed.

After implanting and establishing the parallelism of the needles, their desired spacing is maintained by slipping perforated small

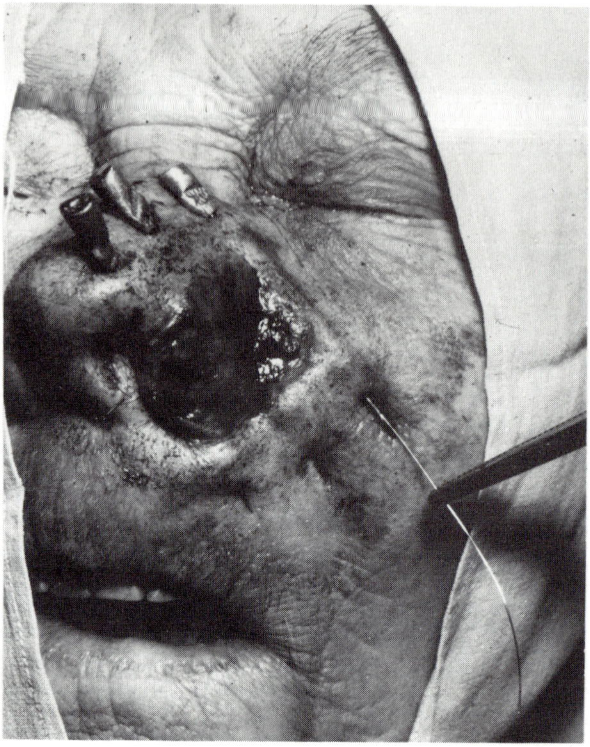

Figure 12. Hypodermic needle technique. Left ala nasi.
a. Direct afterloading of hypodermic needle with I^{192} wire.

segments of lucite or IV tubing over the ends which are then fixed on one side by crushing a lead cap on the bevel of the needle.

Iridium 192 wires are introduced via the other open end with long forceps until only a small segment is visible.

Final insertion of each radioactive wire is accomplished using a special stylet to push the wire into the hypodermic needle until it is well positioned in the target volume.

To complete the setup, the spacing material is slipped over the ends of the needles and lead caps are crushed into place (Figure 12 (b)).

During the loading process, mobile lead screens 2 cm thick are interposed between the operator and the patient to reduce the radiation exposure to the operator and to the assistants (Figure 13).

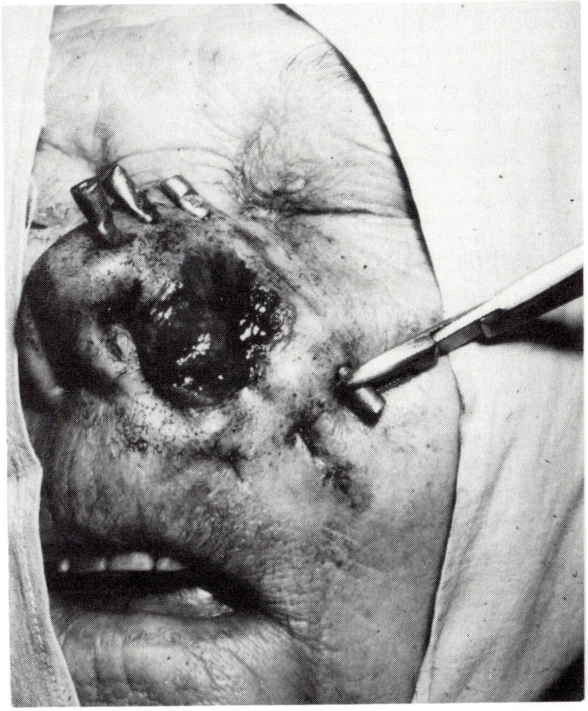

Figure 12
b. Occlusion and immobilization of hypodermic needles with lead caps.

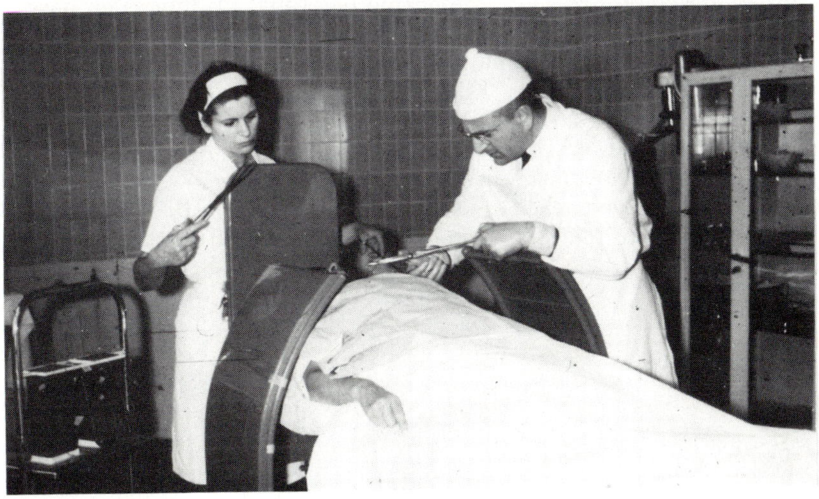

Figure 13. Portable lead screens in position during afterloading phase.

4) Silk Thread Technique

In this technique, Iridium 192 wires are loaded directly into the center of braided silk suture which can then be directly sewn into the desired positions [6]. (see Chapter IX).

5) Cesium 137 Seed Technique (Chassagne's Technique)

General indications:

Plesiotherapy

Uterus and vagina

All target volumes

The reader is referred to the chapter on Gynecology for a detailed description of this technique.

REFERENCES

1. Piérquin, B., Chassagne, D., Gasiorowski, M.: Présentation téchnique et dosimétrique de curiepuncture par fils d'Or 198, *Journal de Radiologie, 40:*690-693, 1959.
2. Hennschke, U., Hilaris, B.S., Mahan, G.D.: Afterloading in interstitial and intracavitary radiation therapy, *Amer. Journal of Roentgenology, 90:*386-395, 1963.
3. Raynal, M., Chassagne, D., Piérquin, B: Utilisation d'un mandrin plastique dans la téchnique d'endocuriethérapie par tubes plastiques, *Annales de Radiologie, 8:*393-396, 1965.
4. Pierquin, B.: Endo et plésioradiothérapie par Iridium 192 et Césium 137, *Radiol. Clin. Biol., 35:*407-418, 1966.
5. Sahatchiev, A., Mouchmov, M.: L'emploi des fils de soie radioactifs dans la téchnique de brachyradiothérapie par tubes plastiques en boucles, *Annales de Radiologie, 14:*491-495, 1971.
6. D. Chassagne, N. Mouchmov, A. Sahatchiev, B. Piérquin: Téchnique D'Endocuriethérapie Par Fils De Soie Radioactifs Dans Les Epithéliomas Cutune's. *Journal Radiol., 54:869-871. 1973.*
7. D. Chassagne: Low-Dose-Rate Technique of Endocavitary Brachytherapy. *Proc. Royal Soc. Med., 66:*936-938, 1973.
8. D. Chassagne, Delouche G., Rocoplan J. A., Piérquin B.: Déscription Et Premiers Essais Du Curietron. *J. Radiol., 50:*910-913, 1969.

Chapter V

DOSIMETRY

In this chapter, we will successively review the dosimetry of photon emitters including Iridium 192 and Cesium 137 and of the beta emitters such as Phosphorus 32, Strontium 90 and Yttrium 90.

DOSIMETRY OF PHOTONS

This dosimetric study is essentially based on our new Paris System (formerly Relational System). We will review:

I. The fundamental characteristics of dose distribution.
II. The rules of the Paris System.
III. Dosimetric planning.
IV. Dosimetric control

I. The Fundamental Characteristics of Dose Distribution

It is essential from the beginning to become aware of the particular conditions of dose distribution in brachytherapy. Unlike teletherapy where the radiation source is at a distance from the tumor and the dose is more homogenously distributed in the target volume, in brachytherapy the sources are within the tumor and the dose at different points in the target volume is distributed most unevenly. The dose is very high at points in contact with the radioactive source, but it drops rapidly at a few mm distance (Figure 14). This variation of dose within and around the target volume is strictly dependent on the geometric dispersion of radiations. In brachytherapy with either Iridium 192 or Cesium 137 the attenuation of photons is of much less importance because of the short target distances involved, usually not exceeding several cm.

The calculation of the dose can be accomplished at one or several points in space or along isodose surfaces.

a. The calculation of the dose at a point in space is an elementary exercise, the classical formulae for which we would like to recall.

For a point radioactive source, or one that could be considered as such at the distance where the dose is determined, the calculation calls simply for the application of the inverse square law. At a point

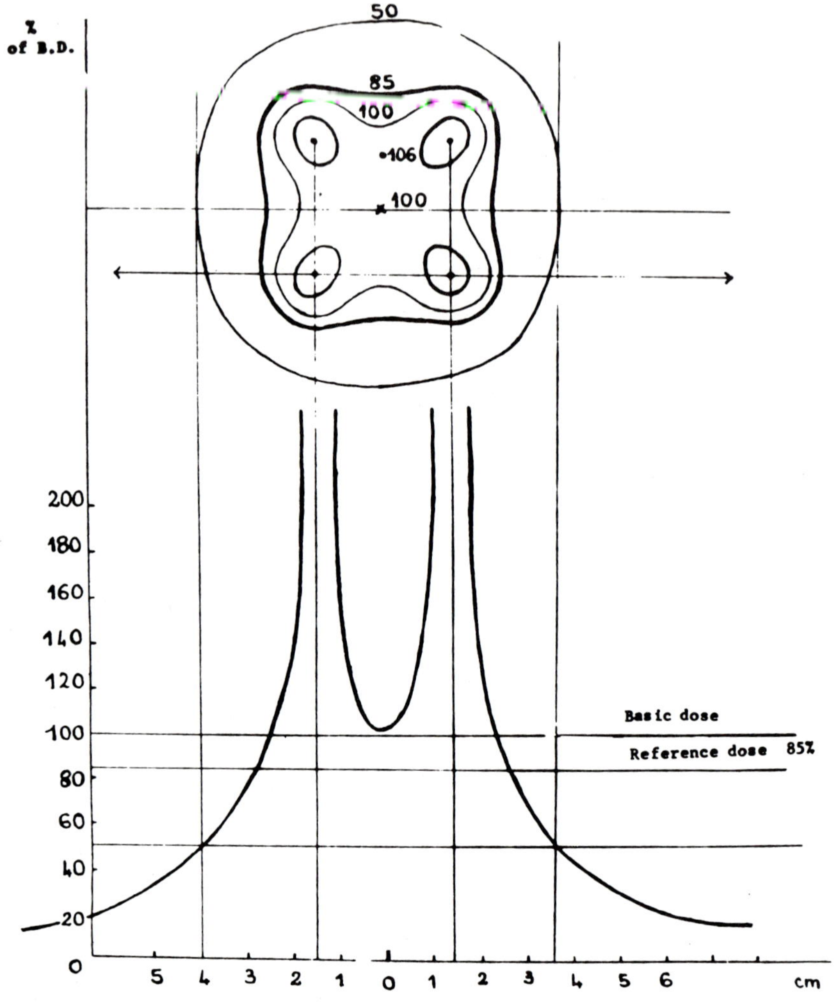

Figure 14. Dose distribution in a target volume implanted with 4 parallel radioactive sources. Cross section and vertical section.

X cm distant from a point source containing Q mCi of a radioactive element with an exposure rate constant Γ, the dose delivered is established by the following formula:

$$D = \Gamma \times \frac{Q}{X^2} \times t$$

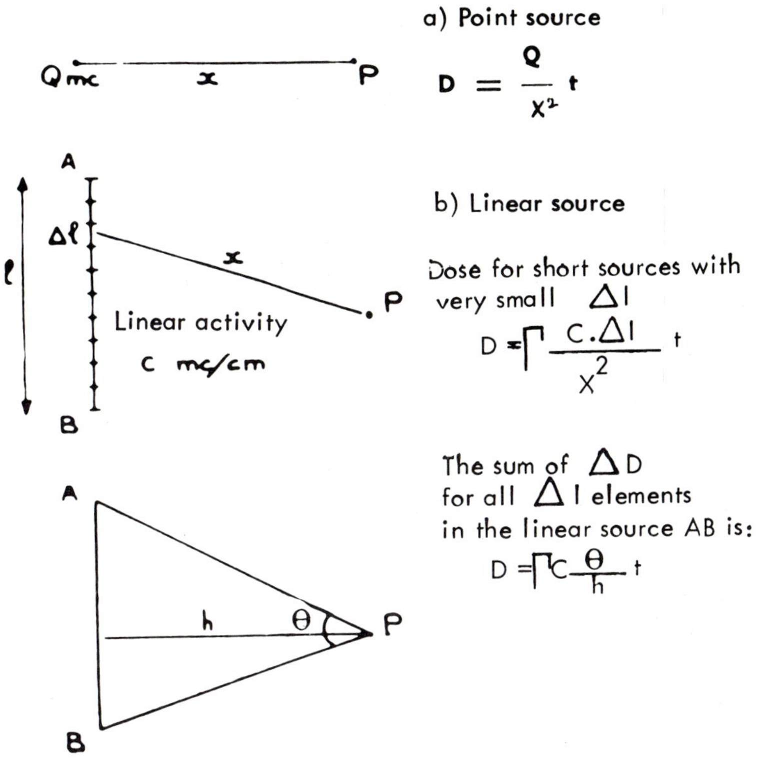

Figure 15 a.b. Calculation of the dose from a point source (a) and from a linear source (b).

While for a linear source AB at point P, h cm distant from the axis of the source, the dose delivered is established by the following formula:

$$D = \Gamma \times C \times \frac{\theta}{h} \times t$$

Where "t" is the duration of the application in hours (Figure 15a). Γ and t are as noted above, the dose factor and the duration of the application respectively. C represents the "linear activity" of the source in mCi/cm where theta is the angle with which point P sees source AB (Figure 15b).

In the case of several linear straight sources, a point in space receives the total of the dose delivered by each source calculated with the above formula.

When there are sources of different types and oriented in different planes, it is still theoretically possible to add the individual doses delivered by each source at any point in space. In reality the calculation is difficult and implies the accurate localization and identification of each source, a very complex task.

b. The calculation of the dose at several different points for the determination of isodose curves.

Irrespective of the type of radioactive material, the calculation of the same dose at several different points, or the determination of isodose curves, is based on complex calculations. To make a detailed study of the dose distribution in and around a target volume, elaborate techniques are essential using either standard isodoses or computers.

These elaborate techniques are the ones commonly used in the actual practice of brachytherapy.

II Rules of the "Paris System"

These rules are based on the fundamental concept of flexible relationships between the length of radioactive sources and their spacing (1,2). Before discussing them, it will be helpful to recall certain clinical factors and to define certain terms.

Tumor volume: Volume of clinically apparent tumor.

Target volume: Tumor volume, plus an additional margin of potentially involved surrounding normal tissue.

Treated volume: Volume of tissue receiving the minimum tumor dose.

Irradiated volume: All the above, plus the surrounding normal tissues encompassed by an isodose having 50% of the value of the reference isodose.

Active length: Length of the radioactive segment of the source.

Separation: The distance between sources, usually ranging from 5 to 22 mm.

Basal dose (B.D.): The minimal dose or the average of several minimal doses at points inside the perimeter formed by the most exterior sources of an implant.

Reference isodose (R. I.): The isodose line corresponding to the treated volume. Its value is 85% of the basal dose. The minimum tumor dose is therefore the reference isodose.

High dose volume (2 R. I.): The isodose with a value twice that of the reference isodose. It includes the areas of high dosage immediately surrounding each radioactive source.

The Rules

1. The radioactive material should be arranged in parallel and straight lines when possible. The direction of these lines defines the axis of implantation. Spacing between the different parallel sources should be as uniform as possible. Anatomy in certain areas will impose variations and produce curved lines, curls and nonparallel setups, such as triangles, which deserve special considerations.

2. Continuity of the radioactive lines is indispensable in order to assure clinical and dosimetric control of the radioactive setup. Such continuity is accomplished either by using continuous radioactive wires, such as Iridium 192, or an easily identifiable continuous framework such as Cesium 137 seed carriers. These methods permit visualization of each radioactive line with image amplifier radiography, standard radiography or tomography.

3. Each radioactive source should extend beyond the limits of the tumor volume so that the minimal dose calculated at the reference isodose is attained over the entire area of the selected target volume. In practice, this requires that radioactive wires protrude in each direction beyond the limits of the target volume, for a distance determined by the relation in size between the treated volume and the radioactive setup (*see* "Dosimetric Planning").

4. The spacing of sources will vary, according to the size of the target volume, within the following limits: 5-10 mm. for a very small volume to 15-22 mm. for a very large volume. These variations are necessary because of the differences in the positions of the isodose lines around wires of different lengths (Figure 16).

5. The spacing of sources must also take into consideration the tolerance to radiation of different tissues. The lower the tolerance, the smaller the separation between radioactive lines, in order to reduce the size of the high-dose volume in the immediate neighborhood of the radioactive wire. The diameter of this high-dose volume should never exceed 1 cm.

6. The length of each radioactive wire is measured according to the exact requirements of the implant.

7. For straight parallel lines, calculation of the dose is made in a

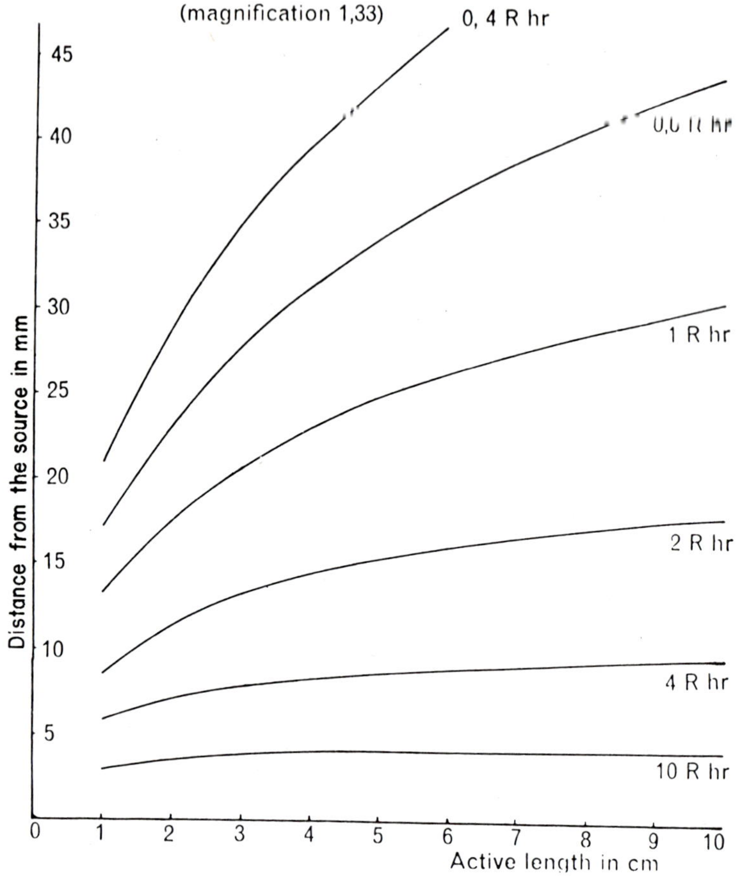

Figure 16. Calibration graphs demonstrating the increase in radius of isodose circles around linear sources of increasing length. The relatively slight increase in the diameter of isodose circles close to the sources explains why long linear sources can be more widely spaced without dangerously increasing the diameter of the high dose zone around the source.

single plane perpendicular to the axis of implantation, passing through the center of the treated volume.

8. After 3-dimensional reconstruction or tomography, this plane shows each radioactive wire as a point (Figure 17). The dose is calculated in the plane of the cross section by applying the "escargot" isodose technique to each point of the tumor under study. (*See* Dosimetric Planning.)

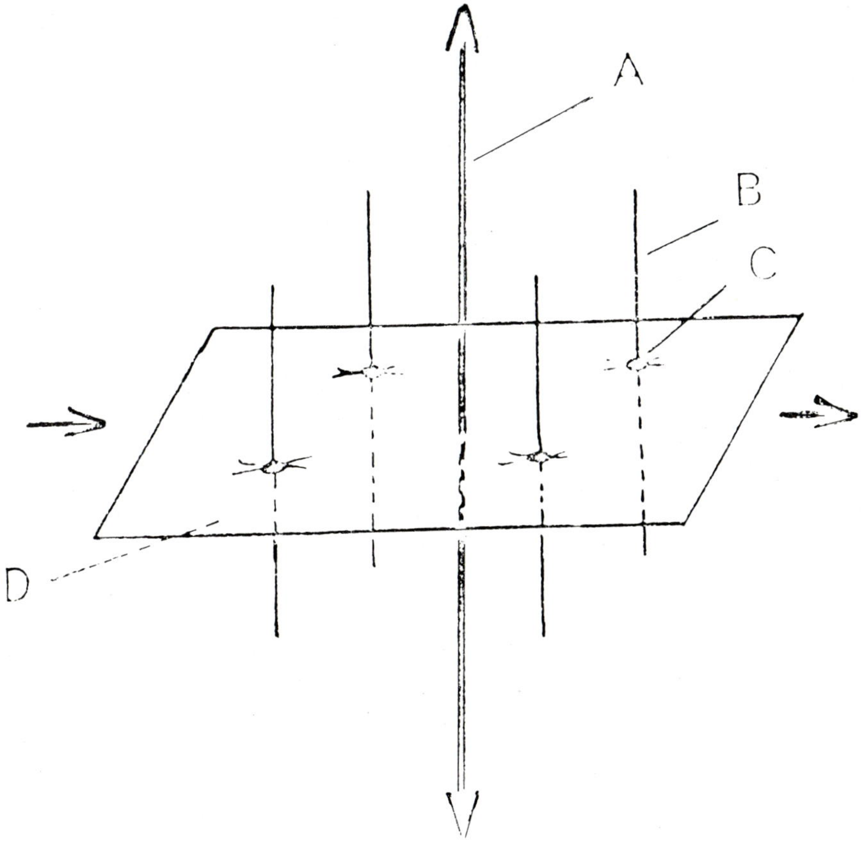

Figure 17. The tomographic plane (D) is oriented perpendicularly to the axis of implantation (A) of the sources (B) which will appear on the tomogram as a small radiopaque point (C).

9. For a volume implant with perfect geometry, the basal dose rate is calculated at points equidistant between adjacent sources (Figure 18). Points on the periphery of the treated volume receiving the same dose rates are identified and continuous lines joining them can be drawn, forming isodoses around the tumor volume (Figure 19 (a,b).

The most useful of these is the reference isodose. Its value is 85 per cent of that of the lowest average dose within the tumor, and it delineates the treated volume.

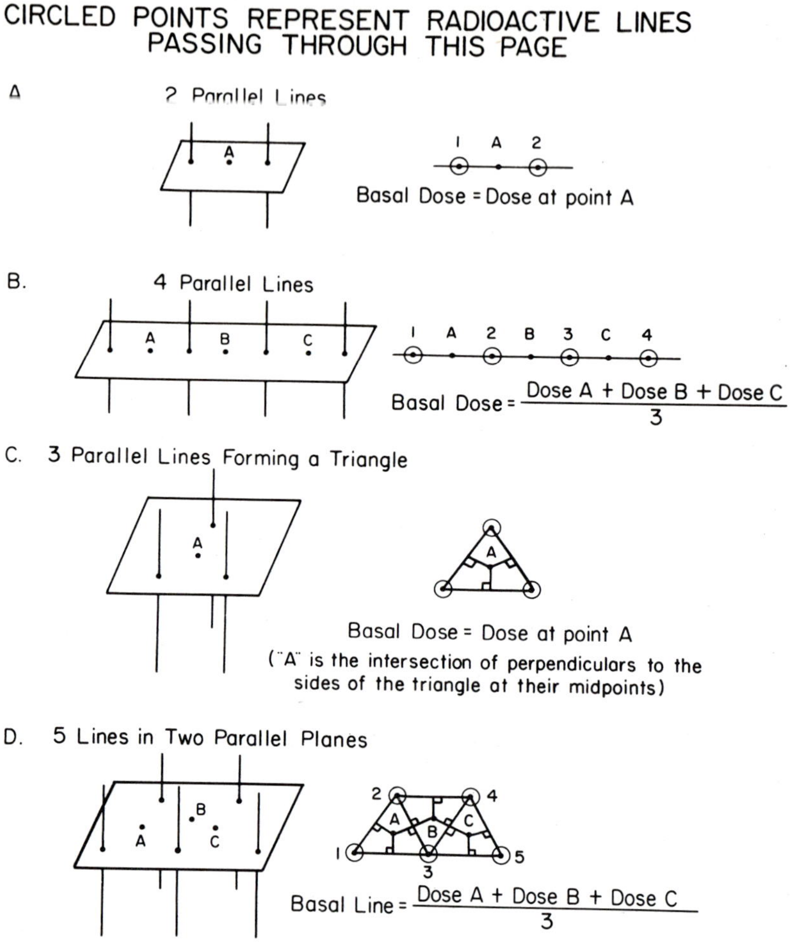

Figure 18. Calculation of basal dose (B.D.)
As shown when the implant is in more than one plane the implanted area is divided into small triangles or rectangles for the calculation of B. D. which is then the average of the B. D. in each section.

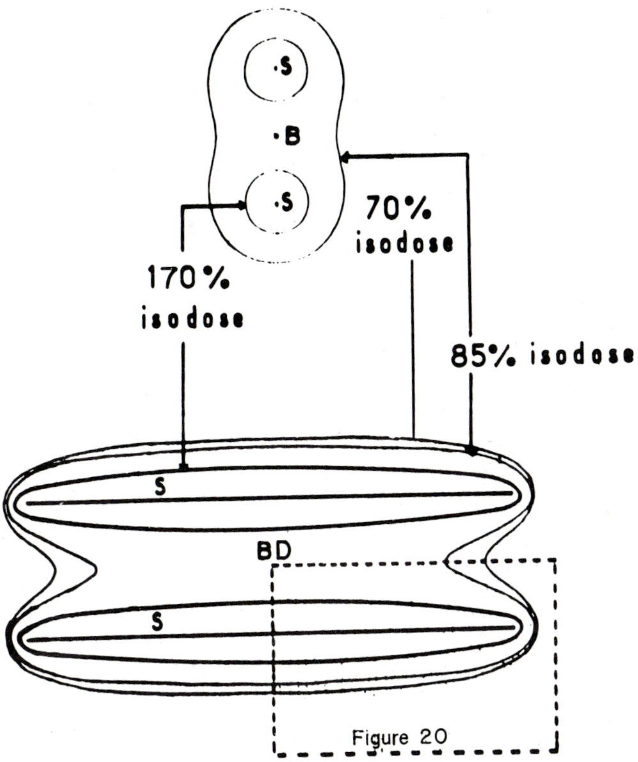

Figure 19. a. Diagram of the relative positions of the reference isodose R. I. = 85% of basal dose (B. D.) and of the high dose volume (2 R. I.) surrounding 2 parallel linear sources.

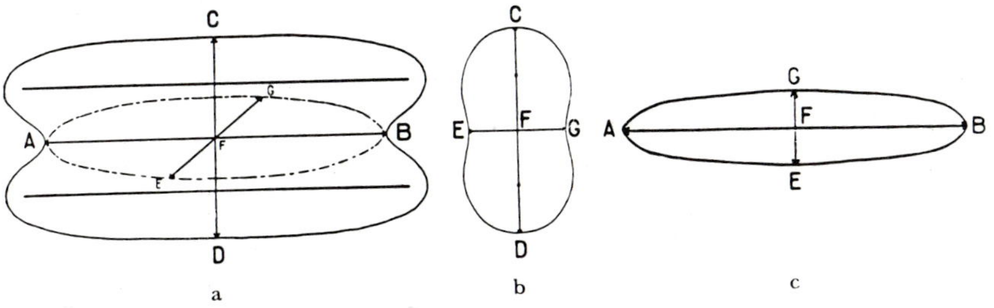

Figure 19. b. Treated volume defined by the reference isodose in 3 planes: a. in the plane of the sources. b. in cross section and c. lateral plane.

Length (AB), Width (CD) and thickness (EG) of the treated volume are indicated.

10. The linear activity of the radioactive material in all wires within a given treated volume is constant. In large treated volumes, correct spacing of lines of equal linear activity gives a dose in the middle of the implant somewhat higher than at the edges. This central boost is generally favorable. Otherwise, it is always possible after appropriate calculations to remove part of the radioactive material from the center of the volume during the course of irradiation, if necessary.

11. Linear activity is normally chosen so that the tumor dose rate (reference isodose) is 30 to 60 rads/hour (about 750 to 1,500 rads/day).

12. Although one cannot fix a rigid upper limit of tumor dose, we usually do not exceed 6,500 rads for a lesion treated solely by endotherapy or plesiotherapy.

13. Biological considerations in a large treatment volume (integral dose) impose an upper safety limit of the total quantity of radioactive material used. In the case of Iridium 192, we do not exceed 150 mCi, and 200 mCi, for Cesium 137 for a six-day treatment.

The establishment of these rules has enabled us to standardize the dosimetric planning.

III. The Dosimetric Planning

Dosimetric planning consists of determining, before the after-loading and in consideration of the dimensions of the target volume, the radioactive setup best assuring an optimal dose distribution in the treated volume.

In order to accomplish this goal, and with the help of computers, we have been able to establish fundamental relationships between the treated volume and the radioactive material for different applications [4] (Figure 20).

A. Single Plane Applications (see Figure 19 (b)).

The three dimensions of the treated volume are:

Length (L) of the treated volume. This is the distance between the boundaries of the treated volume on an axis parallel and equidistant from the two lateral-most radioactive sources. This line is in the plane of the sources and bisects the central corridor of irradiation.

The term "corridor" corresponds to the space between two parallel radioactive sources (Figure 21).

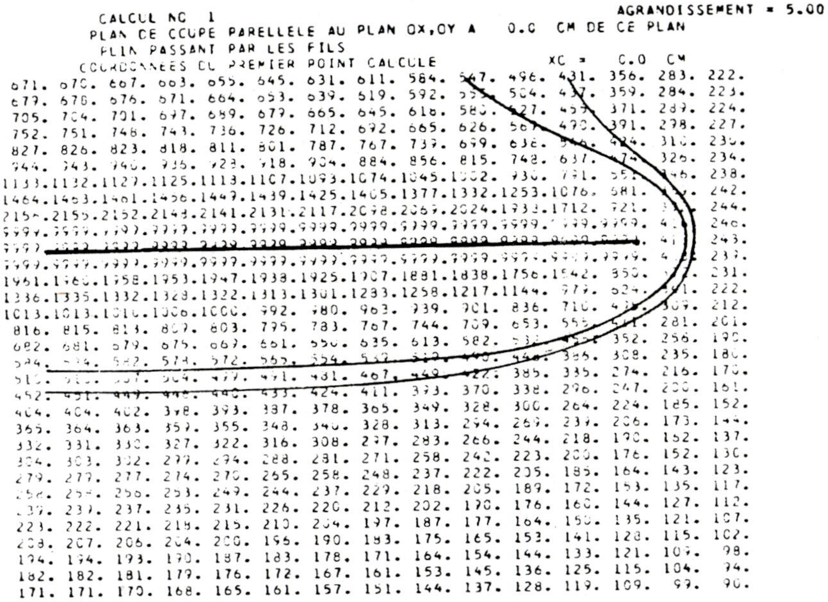

Figure 20. Example of computer calculation sheet showing isodoses in the plane of the sources. The isodose lines surrounding sources are symmetrical therefore it is sufficient to display only the portion shown.

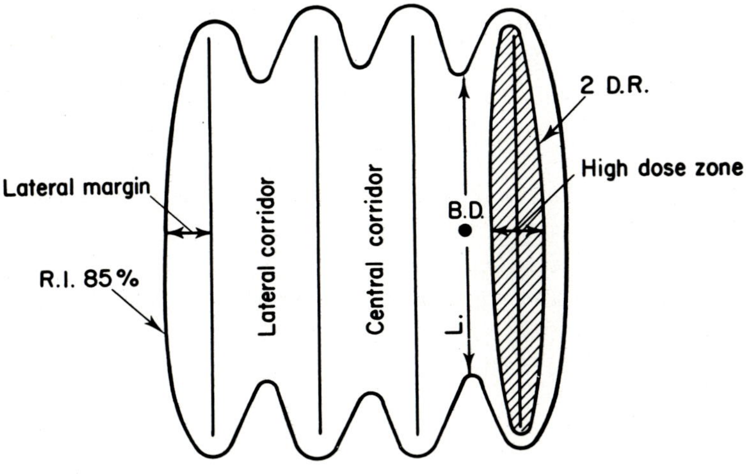

Figure 21. The treated volume around 4 parallel radioactive lines. B.D. basal dosage point L= length of treated volume.

In a setup containing 2 radioactive lines, there is only 1 central corridor.

In a setup with 3 radioactive lines, there are 2 lateral corridors.

In a setup with 4 radioactive lines, there is 1 central and 2 lateral corridors.

In a setup of 5 radioactive lines, there are 2 central and 2 lateral corridors.

In a setup of 6 radioactive lines, there is 1 central corridor, 2 intermediate corridors and 2 lateral corridors.

Thickness (T) of the treated volume. This is the distance between the boundaries of the treated volume on an axis equidistant from the two lateralmost radioactive sources and perpendicular to that axis at its center.

Width (W) of the treated volume. It is the distance between the boundaries of the treated volume on the axis perpendicular to the center of the radioactive sources and in the plane of these radioactive sources.

One can also define a segment of the width that is common to all radioactive setups in one plane, namely the "lateral margin" which is that fraction of the width situated between one of the lateral-most radioactive lines and the reference isodose (Figure 21).

1. Dosimetric Studies of Two Radioactive Lines

a. Relationship between the treated volume and the radioactive material: The dimensions of the treated volume have a simple relationship to the geometry of the radioactive material. Its length depends on the length of the radioactive material, while its width and thickness depend on the spacing of the sources.

(1) The relationship between the length of the treated volume and that of the radioactive materials is given below.

$$\frac{\text{Length of treated volume}}{\text{Radioactive length}} = 0.7$$

This ratio increases slightly when the radioactive lengths increase from 1 to 10 cm.: 0.65 to 0.75 for R. I. 85%.

The length of the treated volume is practically independent of the spacing.

(2) The relationship of the width of the treated volume to the spacing of the radioactive material is as follows:

$$\frac{\text{Width of the treated volume}}{\text{Spacing}} = 1.75$$

For the lateral margin, the following ratio is valid:

$$\frac{\text{Width of the lateral margin}}{\text{Spacing}} = 0.37$$

The width is practically independent of radioactive length for the same spacing.

(3) The relationship between the thickness of the treated volume and the radioactive material is:

$$\frac{\text{Thickness of the treated volume}}{\text{Spacing}} = 0.5$$

These ratios are slightly larger when the radioactive lengths increase from 1 to 10 cm; 0.46 to 0.59 for R. I. 85%.

b. Relationships Within the Treated Volume

(1) Width and Thickness

$$\frac{\text{Width}}{\text{Thickness}} = 3.5$$

These ratios vary moderately when the radioactive lengths vary from 1 to 10 cm: 3.9 to 3 for R. I. 85%.

(2) Length and Width

For small radioactive lengths, the width is numerically larger than the length. For longer radioactive lengths, the length is numerically larger than the width.

There is a transitional zone where the lengths and the widths are equal (see Table I).

TABLE I

Radioactive lengths for which the length and width of treated volumes are equal (in cm)	*:Spacing (in cm) R.I. 85%*
2.5	1.5
3	1.8

(3) Thickness and Diameter of the High Dose Volumes

For the 85% reference isodose, the thickness of the treated volume increases by a factor of 2.3 when the radioactive length increases from 1 to 10 cm while the diameter of the high dose volume (2 R. I.) under these conditions is increased by only a factor of 1.3.

2. Dosimetric Studies of One Radioactive Line

For a single radioactive source, the basal dose is no longer valid. The relationship between the radioactive setup and the treated volume is, therefore, established only by analogy with those already discussed for two radioactive sources.

Only two dimensions of the treated volume can be studied:

The width which is identical to the thickness.

The length which is along the axis of the radioactive source itself.

a. Width of the Treated Volume

Only the maximum width of the treated volume is defined in relation to the active length. Based on the maximum acceptable dimensions of the area of the high dose volume, we recommend limiting the width of the treated volume as described in Table II (Figures 22 and 23).

TABLE II

Radioactive Length (in cm)	*Width of Treated Volume* (in cm)
1	0.9
2	1.2
3	1.3
4	1.4
5	1.4
6	1.5
7	1.5
8	1.5
9	1.6
10	1.6

b. Length of the Treated Volume (Figure 24).

Situated along the axis of the radioactive source, the length of the treated volume projects well beyond the boundaries of the

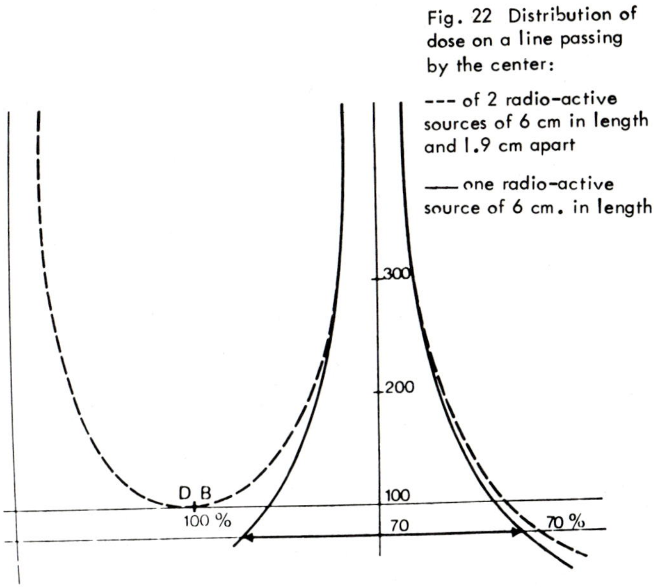

Figure 22. Dose distribution on a plane passing through the center of two radioactive sources, 6 cm long and spaced by 1.9 cm vs one radioactive source 6 cm long.

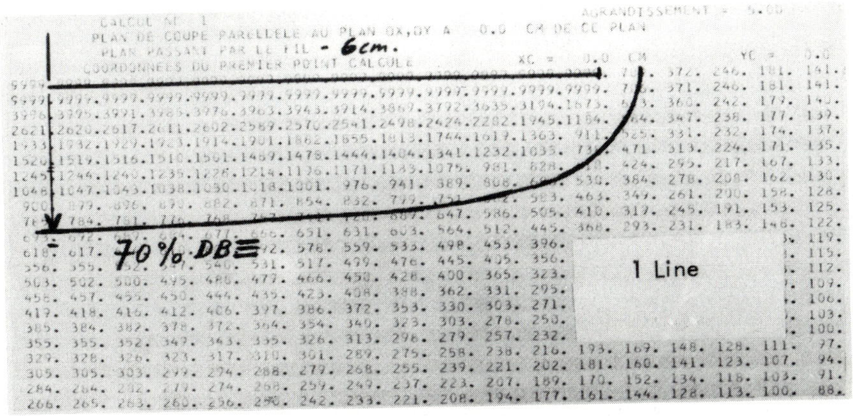

Figure 23. Computer dosimetric study of single source 6 cm long. The isodose lines correspond by analogy to those for 2 parallel sources of the same length with maximal spacing. 70% isodose depicted.

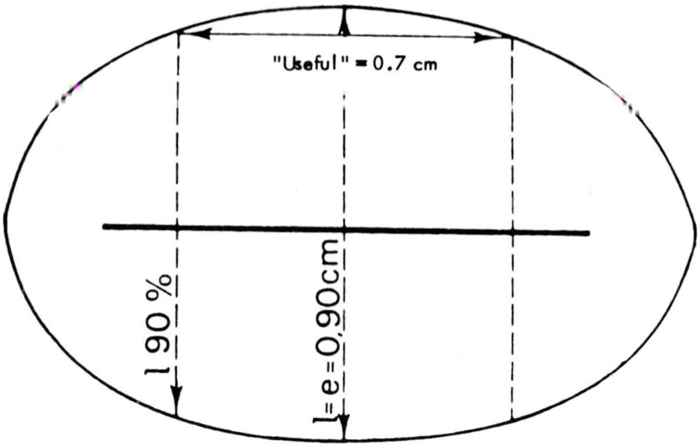

Figure 24. Dosimetric study of a single linear source 1 cm in length. "Useful" length indicated.

radioactive length. It is, therefore, necessary to define a "useful length" which is equal to:

$$\frac{\text{"Useful" length}}{\text{Radioactive length}} = 0.7$$

3. Dosimetric Study of Three, Four and Five Radioactive Lines

For more than two radioactive lines, the basal dose is defined as the mean of the basal doses determined in each of the corridors of radiation. The other definitions remain valid.

The relationships between the treated volume and the radioactive material described for two radioactive lines can be transposed with slight variations as follows (Figures 25 and 26):

-The ratio $\frac{\text{length of treated volume}}{\text{active length}}$ is practically identical to that for two sources, equalling 0.7

-The ratio $\frac{\text{lateral margin}}{\text{spacing}}$ is slightly less than that for two sources, namely 0.34 instead of 0.37

-The ratio $\frac{\text{thickness}}{\text{spacing}}$ is slightly larger than that for two sources, or 0.6 instead of 0.5

These percentages have been calculated in the lateral corridors of irradiation. For the central corridors, they should be increased by 8

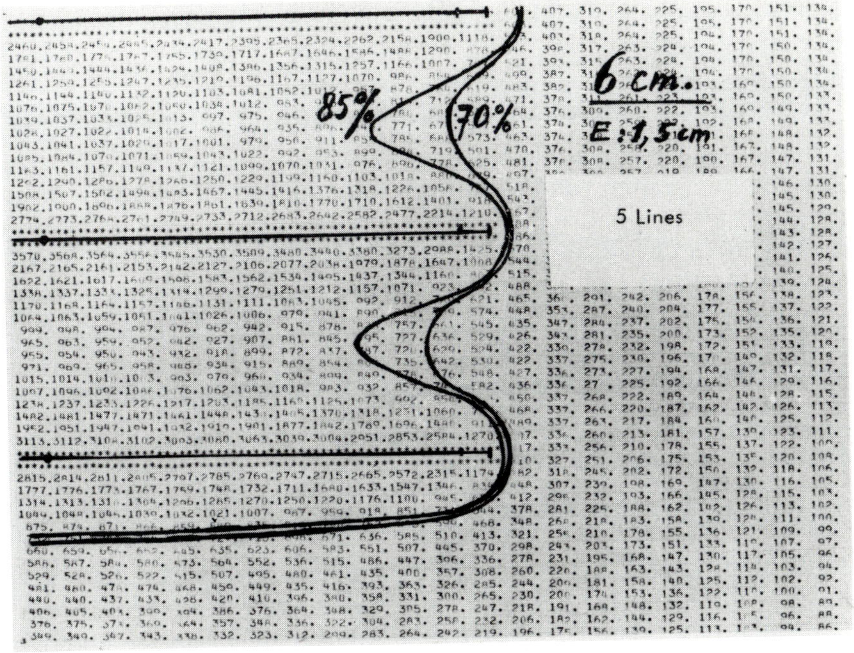

Figure 25. Computer study of 5 parallel sources 6 cm long and spaced by 1.5 cm Dosimetry in same plane as sources.

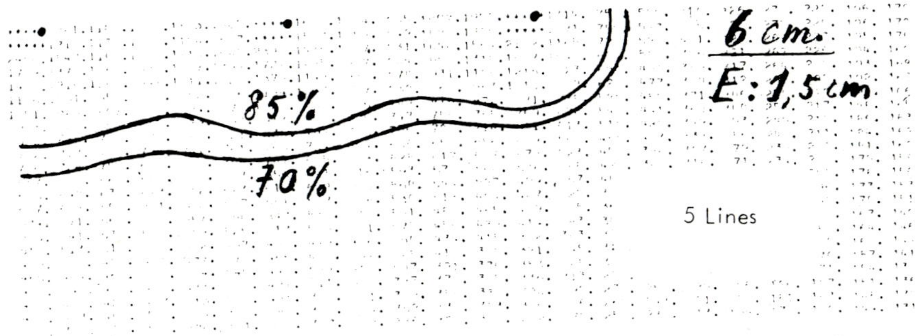

Figure 26. Computer study of 5 parallel sources (Figure 25) Dosimetry in plane perpendicular to the sources at their center.

to 10% for the length of the treated volume and by about 5% for the thickness.

B. Radioactive Applications in Several Planes

The study of radioactive applications in two or three planes of straight and parallel lines confirms the validity of the relationships between the treated volume and the radioactive material. The dose at equidistant points in the central corridors can be greater by as much as 10 to 15% as compared with the dose calculated in the lateral corridors. This augmentation is acceptable and may be favorable considering that the central zone of the target volume is where the least vascularized and the least radiosensitive part of the tumor is located.

In conclusion, according to the principles of the Paris system, the longer the radioactive sources, the greater the spacing.

Three factors justify this statement:

1. Physically, the diameter of the high dose volume surrounding a radioactive source increases proportionally less as the distance between the radioactive source and the reference isodose increases.

2. Technically, in view of the difficulty of assuring a strict parallelism of the longer sources, the risk of creating hot or cold spots becomes greater with very small spacings.

3. Clinically, the thickness is usually greater for longer target volumes.

We have, however, established an upper limit of 2.2 cm spacing, corresponding to a maximum diameter of the high dose volume of approximately 1 cm around sources 10 cm in length.

Radioactive lengths between 1 and 10 cm are used clinically. It is conceivable to plan applications with longer radioactive sources and not increase the maximum spacing of 2.2 cm.

In consideration of the dose rates and the duration of the application, it is important to recognize the relationship between the basal dose and the spacing of radioactive sources of different lengths.

Table III summarizes these relationships:

TABLE III

Iridium 192. Linear Activity of 1 mCi/cm

Radioactive length in cm (activity = 1 mCi/cm)	*Spacing Between 2 Parallel Lines in cm*			
1	0.8	0.9	1	1.1
2	1.1	1.2	1.3	1.4
3	1.2	1.3	1.4	1.6
4	1.2	1.3	1.5	1.7
5	1.3	1.4	1.6	1.8
6	1.3	1.4	1.6	1.9
7	1.3	1.5	1.7	1.9
8	1.3	1.5	1.7	2
9	1.3	1.5	1.7	2
10	1.3	1.5	1.8	2.1
B. D. in rad/hr	40	35	30	25

A provisional atlas of different radioactive setups with straight and parallel sources is presently under study (Figure 27).

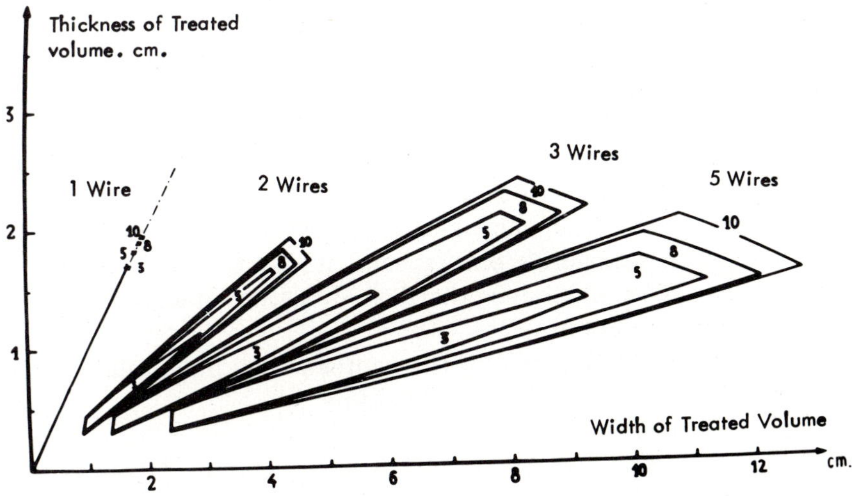

Figure 27. Diagram for evaluating the number of wires to be used as function of the dimensions of the volume to be treated. WAMBERSIE *et al.* (6)

C. Special Considerations

1. Cylindrical Volumes of Straight and Parallel Radioactive Sources

On a single circumference, we recommend using not more than five radioactive sources forming a pentagon. With maximum spacing of 2.1 cm between each source, this gives a treated volume which resembles a cylinder with a diameter of 4 cm within the boundaries of the 85% reference isodose (Figure 28).

2. Curved Treated Volume with Curved and Parallel Sources

In such applications, the dose distribution is asymmetrical, being higher on the concave side. For an arc less than 30°, the dose should be corrected. This is best accomplished by computer.

3. Loops

The curved portion of the apex of a loop should be considered as divided into two parts and the length of each half added to the overall length of either side.

4. Triangular Volumes

In certain cases, it may be necessary to encompass a lesion with three radioactive sources forming an equilateral triangle. In order not to exceed the margins of permissible high dose, the sides of the triangle should be less than 4 cm in length. The points of intersection should be left inactive to avoid hot spots (Figure 29).

The basal dose can be calculated at the center of this setup with the use of escargot isodoses. However, a detailed calculation of dose cannot be well established, particularly the reference isodose, except by computer.

5. Volume Treated with Radioactive Pins

In view of the frequency and the importance of the clinical application of radioactive pins, special study of their dosimetry is imperative. We will discuss the dose distribution surrounding a hairpin and simple pin.

a. Dosimetry at the level of the center of the pins: relationship between the pins and the treated volume.

1) Hair Pin (Figure 30 (a, b))

Based on a standard linear activity of 1 mCi/cm, the basal dose varies according to the length of the pin and is about 40 rads per hour. The length of the treated volume which is measured on a line that is equidistant from and parallel to the branches of the pin,

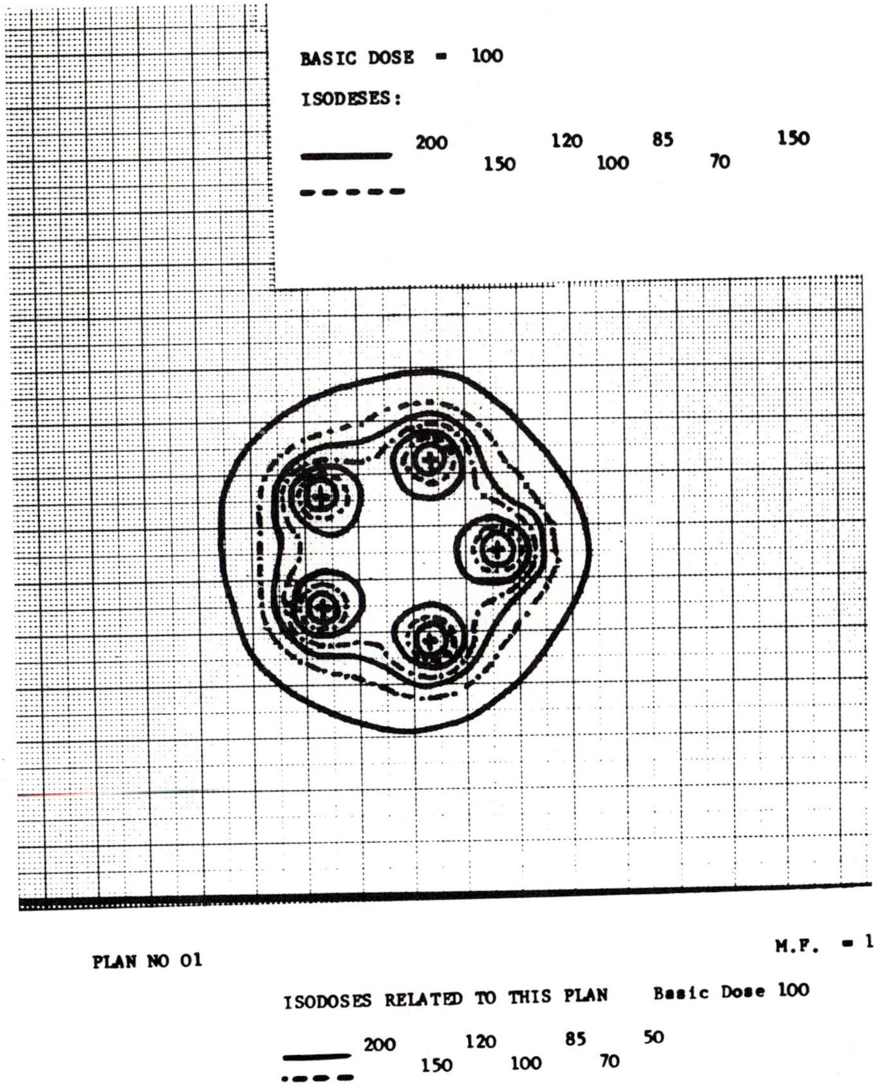

Figure 28. Dose distribution surrounding 5 sources implanted in pentagonal form.

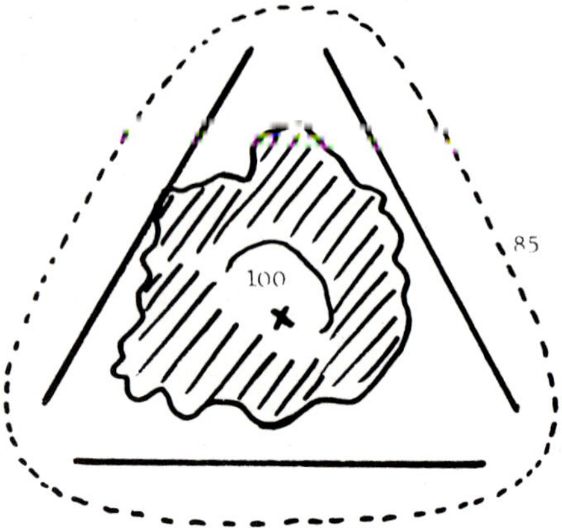

Figure 29. Dose distribution surrounding 3 linear sources forming an equilateral triangle.

extending from the reference isodose at the tip of the pin, and the tangent that crosses the aspices of the "M" of the head, is of the order of 0.75 for the shortest pin (2 em) and 0.8 for the longest pin (5 cm). The width of the treated volume, measured on a line perpendicular to the parallel branches of the pin and crossing the point where the BD is measured, is about 1.66 cm. being nearly identical for the different lengths of the pins used. The thickness of the treated volume related to the spacing is about 0.6 cm. ranging between 0.58 for 2 cm. long pins and 0.66 for 5 cm. pins. Table IV gives the values of these different relationships for different lengths of the hairpins.

TABLE IV

Iridium 192 hairpin linear activity 1 mCi/cm

Length of pin (cm)	*B. D. (Rad/hr.)*	*Length of Treated Volume (cm)*	*Width of Treated Volume Center (cm)*	*Thickness of Treated Volume Center (cm)*
2	36.2	1.5	2.0	0.6
3	38.2	2.4	2.0	0.7
4	39.9	3.3	2.1	0.8
5	41.1	4.2	2.1	0.8

2) Simple Pin (Figure 30 (c)): Refer to dosimetric studies of one radioactive line.

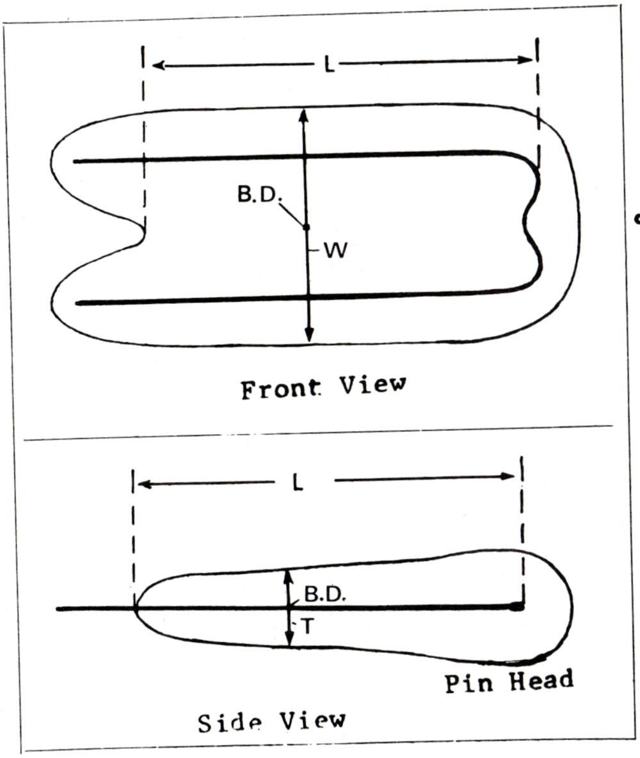

Figure 30. a.b. Reference isodose (85% to B.D.) around a hairpin 4 cm long
B.D. = position of basal dose
L = length of treated volume
Lq = width of treated volume
Ep = thickness of treated volume

b. Dosimetry at the Level of the Heads of the Pins

1) Hairpin

The thickness of the treated volume increases near the transverse branch, while the width diminishes as compared to the center. The reference isodose curves marking the thickness or width are almost parallel to the two branches of the pin in the zone between its head and center (Figure 30 (a, b)).

The following table gives the various values for the width and thickness for the different lengths of hairpins.

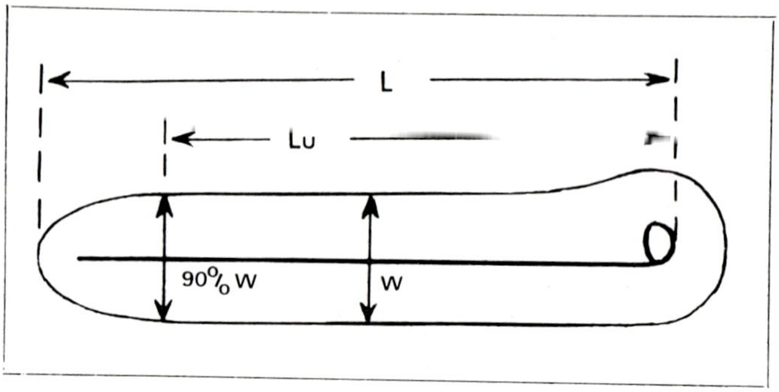

Figure 30. c. Reference isodose around a single pin 4 cm long
L = length of treated volume
W = width of treated volume
Lu = useful length

TABLE V

Dimensions of Treated Volumes for Hairpins

Length of pin (cm)	*Width of treated Volume* Center (cm)	Head	*Thickness of Treated Volume* Center (cm)	Head
2	2.0	1.8	0.6	0.9
3	2.0	1.7	0.7	0.9
4	2.1	1.7	0.8	0.9
5	2.1	1.7	0.8	1.0

On the main axis of the pin, which is equidistant from the two parallel branches and which passes through the center of the transverse branch, the dose drops very rapidly to reach a "plateau" within a few mm from the head (Figure 31).

2) Simple Pin

The width of the reference isodose at the head of the simple pin is practically identical to that at its center. It is, however, slightly deviated to the side of the eyelet in relation to the main axis of the pin. The same is true for the thickness in the case of single pins (Figure 30 (c)).

In summary, the heads of Iridium 192 pins, that is, the transverse branch of the hairpin and the eyelet of the simple pin, serve the purpose of "crossing."

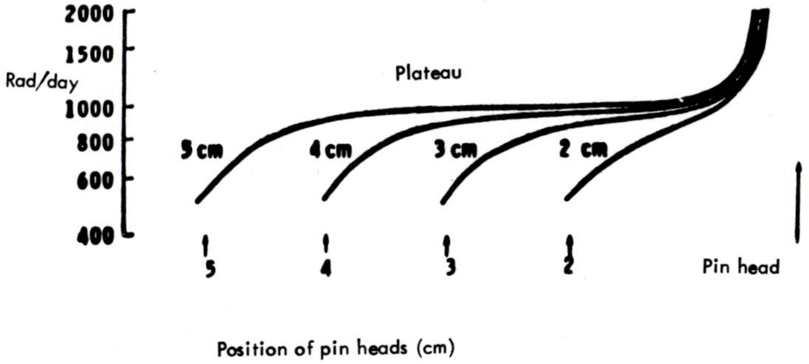

Figure 31. Dose rate along an axis equidistant from the radioactive branches of hairpins 2 to 5 cm in length.

c. Dosimetry at the Tips of the Pins

1) Hairpin

The dimensions of the treated volume diminish rapidly at the tips of the hairpins. (Figure 30 (a, b)) Thickness becomes negligible and the reference isodose sags inwardly by several mm between the two branches. Considering this fact, it is important to define the useful length of the treated volume at a level where the thickness is still significant. We have chosen a level where the thickness is 90% of that calculated at the center (Figure 30 (b)).

Table VI shows the "useful" lengths corresponding to the various lengths of hairpins.

TABLE VI

Useful Lengths of Hairpins

Length of Pin (cm)	*Length of Treated Volume*	*Useful Length of Treated Volume*
2	1.5	1.1
3	2.4	1.8
4	3.3	2.5
5	4.2	3.5

At the ends of the hairpins, the zone of underdosage is appreciable (Figure 31). The radiotherapist should, therefore, choose a radioactive length such that the distal boundary of the treated volume remains enclosed within this "cold zone," by choosing a radioactive length that is about 1/3 longer than the treated volume.

IV. Dosimetric Control

Dosimetric control is the most important part of the dosimetry; for it determines the effective distribution of the dose.

The placement of a rigid material can encounter anatomical difficulties which are unpredictable and result in an application which is quite different from that which was originally planned. It is important to know the different anatomical structures within the tumor, as well as in the surrounding healthy tissues.

Two methods of control are considered; direct dosimetry via a detector placed in vivo, and indirect dosimetry using roentgenograms to graphically reconstruct the geometry of the implantation.

A. Direct Dosimetry: All methods of calculating the dose based on graphic or material reconstruction of the radioactive setups are involved and delicate, despite the fundamental simplicity of each step. It would be more convenient to obtain a direct measurement of the delivered doses in vivo. There are, however, several technical difficulties which have not yet been overcome. A detector that is introduced directly into the target volume to be irradiated can be inserted and positioned only approximately, because of the rapid fluctuations of dose within the volume. To avoid gross errors in relation to the basal dose or to the reference dose, multiple measurements are necessary. However, multiplicity of measurements can traumatize the patient and may lead to unnecessary radiation exposure of the personnel.

We, therefore, advise against the routine use of direct dosimetry whether by scintillation microdosimeters or by thermoluminescent substances such as lithium fluoride. These techniques, however, may be of value for research purposes.

B. Indirect Dosimetry: Only the following methods presently allow a rigorous control of the dose.

1. Three Dimensional Reconstruction of the Radioactive Setup

Using roentgenograms, the radioactive setup can be spatially reconstructed.

a) Use of Stereographic Images: This method makes use of "reconstruction" instruments by which the geometric configurations are reproduced using moving mobile parts, to locate and establish a point in space based on stereographic projections. An instrument of this type has been described by Mussell.[11]

b) Use of Tomographic Images: The radioactive setup is simultaneously tomographed in four or five evenly spaced planes using an x-ray multicassette unit. These planes are as perpendicular to the axis of implantation as possible. Each film is placed in a multiplane setup corresponding to that of the multicassette and perforated at the location of each radioactive source. A phantom material is used to reconstruct the radioactive setup by passing it through the corresponding performations. Egan and Johnson have constructed such a tomographic setup [13] .

2. Graphic Analysis of the Dose in One or More Planes.

These methods are the ones we recommend and which are very accurate.

For radioactive setups with complicated geometry, we recommend a calculation by computer from orthogonal x rays. Since the initial work of Shalek[15], computer programs for endo- and plesiotherapy have multiplied. The advantages of computer analysis are that the relationships of the isodose curves to the radioactive sources is displayed simultaneously in three or more planes and with calculations of the dose at any desired point. There are existing programs for gynecologic plesiotherapy [17], for curved lines and for any interstitial implant [18].

For radioactive setups involving parallel radioactive sources, we recommend a "point technique" of calculation based on direct measurements or on tomograms.

Point Technique[2]

When dealing with complex structures, it is only natural to think of making a cross section of these structures on a plane perpendicular to the axis of the elements to be analyzed. This is precisely why we have come to study brachytherapeutic dosimetry on cross sections perpendicular to the axis of implantation. When dealing with parallel and continuous radioactive sources, one can obtain cross sectional projections of the radioactive sources either by tomography or by direct measurement when the implantation is superficial enough.

"Escargot" curves are manipulated on these cross sectional displays allowing the calculation of the dose at any point and determination of the location of any isodose line.

We exemplify this technique with a case of squamous cell carcinoma of the mobile portion of the tongue treated by the guide gutter technique of endotherapy (Figure 32 (a, b)).

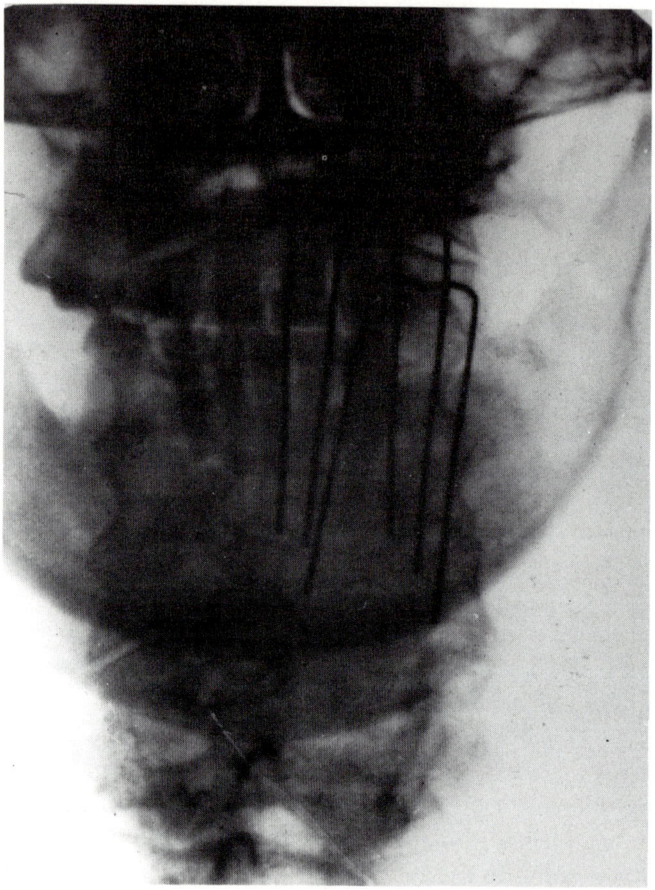

Figure 32. Squamous carcinoma left lateral border of mobile tongue (T_2). Three hairpins 4 cm in length. Dosimetric control.
a. Frontal roentgenogram

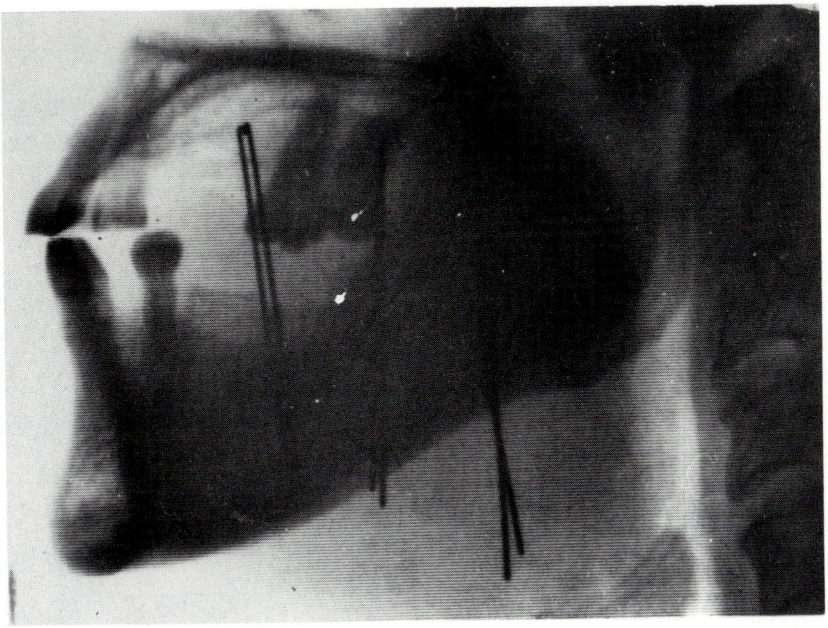

Figure 32. b. Lateral roentgenogram.

Since the implantation has been accomplished in the vertical direction, a transverse axial tomogram is used for the cross sectional studies. The implantation is composed of three hairpins, 4 cm in length giving a total of 6 vertical radioactive liens.

Tomographic Technique

a. Projection of the Axis of Implantation on the Skin

Using a wax pencil, the axis of implantation is drawn on the skin of the patient anteriorly and laterally, using either fluoroscopy or roentgenograms. A line perpendicular to the axis is then drawn on the skin at a level corresponding to the mean center of the radioactive lines. It is at this level that the tomogram will be taken. (Figure 33)

b. Position of the Patient for Tomography

With the patient in the sitting position, the vertical axis is oriented parallel to the axis of rotation of the unit. The horizontal skin line

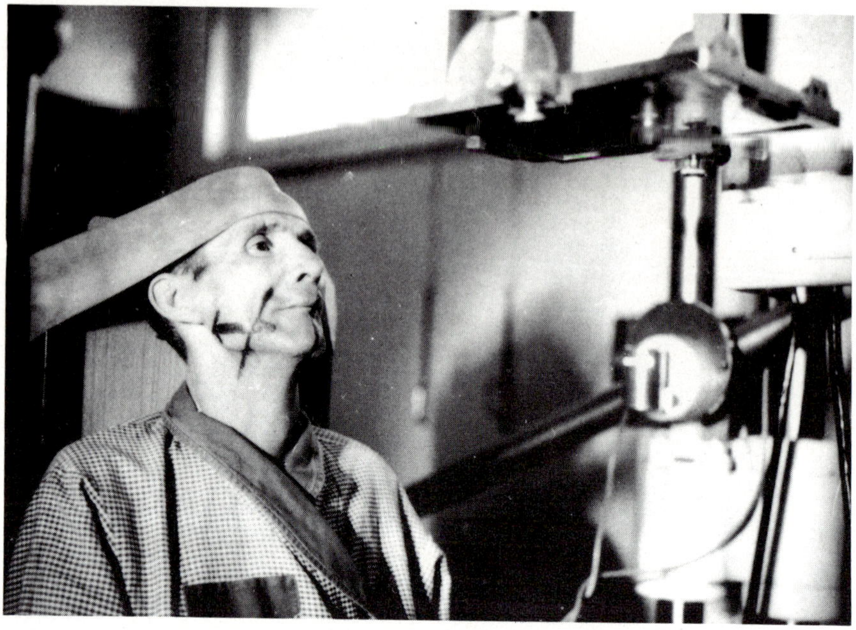

Figure 33. Squamous carcinoma left lateral border of tongue (Figure 32) Patient in position for transverse axial tomography. Note skin marks.

defining the level of the desired cross section is then aligned with the illuminated horizontal plane of the tomogram and the film obtained.

c. Interpreting the Roentgenogram

Six points corresponding to the six radioactive sources will appear on the tomogram (Figure 34).

The anatomic structures are fairly well visualized including the skin contour, the horizontal branches of the mandible, the soft tissue of the pharynx, tongue, the oropharyngeal cavity and the cervical vertebrae. The superimposed image of the brachytherapy setup in one plane is also seen and a tracing of this tomogram can be quickly made.

If the implantation is in a horizontal direction or nearly so, one can use unidirectional tomography (Grossmann or Vallebona movement). According to the requirements of the implantation, the image obtained can be oriented in a sagittal, frontal and intermediate plane. A constant magnification factor should be used. We recommend a factor of 1.33.

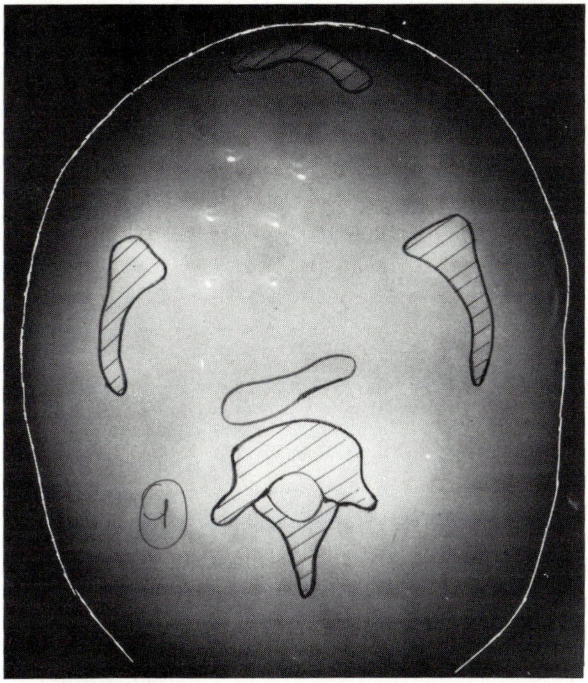

Figure 34. Resultant transverse axial tomogram. Three hairpins seen as 6 opaque points. Anatomic structures have been outlined.

Escargot Technique (Iridium 192)

A tracing of the tomogram is made outlining the important anatomy and the location of the radioactive sources is carefully indicated. The dose is calculated using the "escargot" (Figure 35).

This method is quite satisfactory for implantations with continuous and parallel sources allowing the calculation of isodoses at any level. It should be noted that parallelism between the different radioactive sources is a necessary condition of any good implantation. However, technical and anatomical conditions may exist which will cause an angulation of sources. Angulations of not more than ± 10° result in only negligible variations in the dose in any tomographic plane. With angulation of ± 25°, an error of 10% exists. Deviation from good parallelism may, therefore, require studying the implant at several tomographic levels.

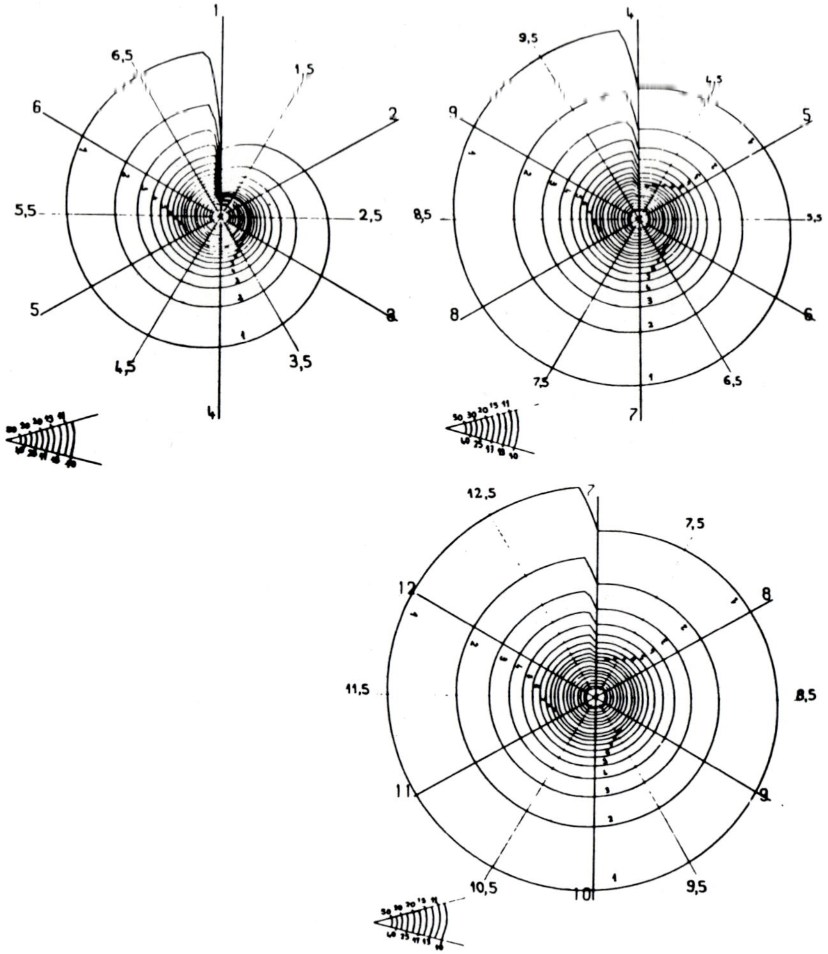

Figure 35. The three "escargot" isodose sheets calculated by computer and drawn with the curve tracer. The values of the isodoses in close proximity to the sources are indicated in the enlarged drawing at the lower left corner of each escargot.

In our point technique system, we use a group of standard isodoses, which unlike circular isodoses that are centered on the radioactive sources are centered on the different points of interest in the tumor. These are the "escargot" isodose curves (10)

In practice, this technique consists of isodoses drawn on transparent sheets of plastic. The first sheet contains the isodoses for radioactive lengths varying between 1 and 6.5 cm; the second one for radioactive lengths from 4.5 to 9.5 cm, and the third is for lengths from 7 to 12.5 cm. The radioactive sources are studied at 0.5 cm intervals. Their layout is similar to wheel spokes around a central axis. By choosing appropriate sheets, this method can be applied to any length of radioactive source in question, whether these lengths are in full cm or not.

There are 19 different isodoses; namely, 50, 40, 30, 25, 20, 17, 15, 13, 11, 10, 9, 8, 7, 6, 5, 4, 3, 2 and 1 rad/hr. for an activity of 1 mCi/cm. The continuous drawing for each value between different radioactive lengths results in isodoses in a helicoidal form resembling a snail, hence the name "escargot"[39].

These isodoses are magnified by a factor of 1.33 corresponding to our magnification factor in tomography.

The calculations are done as follows:

-The reproduction of the tomogram, or the direct measurement, magnified by a factor of 1.33, is attached to a styrofoam pad (Figure 36).

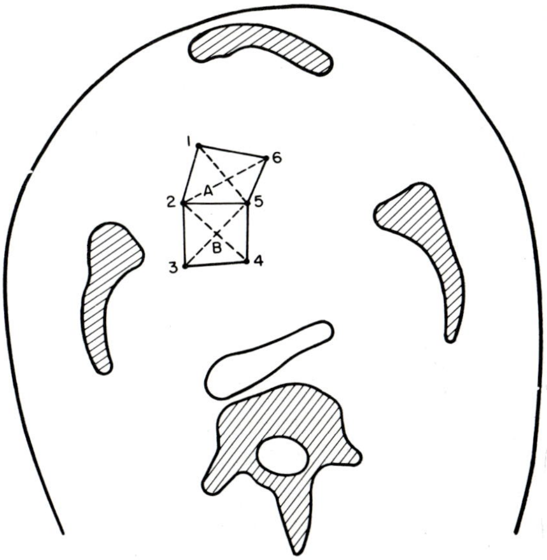

Figure 36. Squamous carcinoma, left lateral border. Dosimetric calculation.

Tracing taken from the transverse axial tomogram (Figure 32-34) Basal dose equals average of basal doses at points A and B using "escargot".

-The appropriate "escargot" is then placed on this drawing by immobilizing its center over any point of interest with a pin which simultaneously perforates the isodose sheet and the drawing, and fixes them to the underlying pad.

-By turning the isodose sheet around this point, one can successively determine the dose contribution to this point from any of the sources (Figure 37).

Source number	Dose rate received by Point A	Dose rate received by Point B
1	12.8	3.9
2	8.5	10.1
3	2.8	12.8
4	4.4	13
5	16	13
6	9.2	3.9
Total	53.7	56.7

$$\text{Basal dose rate} = \frac{53.7 + 56.7}{2}\ \text{rads/hr} = \underline{55.2\ \text{rads/hr}}$$

Figure 37. Sample calculation of basal dose rate in rad/hr. for linear activity 1 m Ci/cm. The dose rate at the minimal dose points A and B from each source is determined from the tomographic tracing using the escargot isodose curves.

-This process can be repeated for multiple points to establish the basal dose and the reference isodose (Figure 38).

-We recommend first calculating the dose at the level of different points of the basal dose, then drawing the boundaries of the desired target volume and finally calculating certain test points on its margins to establish the definitive position of the reference isodose, based on which the total tumor dose is calculated. With a little experience, this dosimetric control can be achieved in only a few minutes.

The escargot technique offers several advantages:

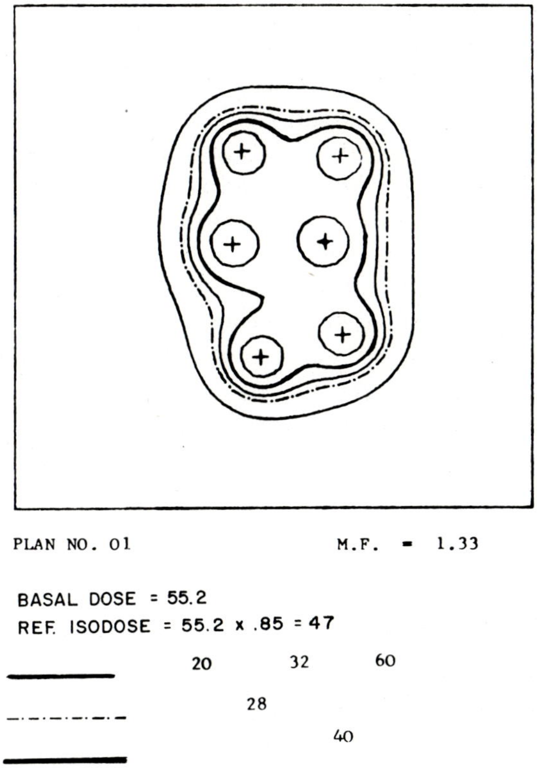

Figure 38. Resultant dose distribution around implant (Fig. 32 a-b). Treated volume defined by reference isodose. In this instance

Reference isodose = 30 rad/hr. for

.85

1. Precision due to the establishment of these isodoses by computers and direct printing by curve tracers.
2. The great number of available values for different radioactive lengths as well as isodoses; in effect, interpolations are reduced to negligible intervals.
3. The large surface of these isodose sheets permits the inclusion of low value isodoses at great distances from the point under study, and can, therefore, be used for large target volumes and can give the dose in peripheral normal tissues.
4. Clarity of reading despite a great number of isodoses.
5. Low cost and compactness.

V. Dosimetry of Electrons

Because beta particles travel short distances of a few mm in tissue, dosimetric problems are quite different as compared to photon therapy. Theoretical calculation is often replaced by direct measurement. In endotherapy, the planning and dosimetric control must consider each of the sources individually because of the very short distances involved. The calculation of the dose should be analyzed in the following instances:

1. In a small target volume implanted with beta emitter seeds. The only case that we practically encounter is that of implantation of the pituitary with several seeds of Yttrium 90. If the seeds are considered as a point source, the calculation is rather simple; the variation of the dose in function of distance is dependent upon the geometric dispersion which introduces a factor of $1\frac{1}{X2}$. There is an extremely high tissue absorption of beta radiation, causing the dose to drop very rapidly.

If the seeds are joined in a sphere or cylinder, the calculation of the dose becomes very complex [4]. In any event, the dose drop off is rapid and the technique allows the satisfactory irradiation of only a few mm of tissue. Several sources are necessary when the target volume acquires a size of more than 1 mm^3.

2. In targets implanted with linear sources of pure beta emitters, for example Yttrium 90 needles [18], we calculate the dose rate at 2 mm from the needle wall. This dose rate is 10 rads per minute for a linear activity of 1 mCi/cm. At more than 4 mm from the wall, the dose is negligible.

For surface applicators of either Phosphorus 32 or Strontium 90, we use the maximum dose rate at the active surface.

REFERENCES

1. Pierquin, B., and Dutreix, A.: Towards a new system in curietherapy (encocurietherapy and plesiocurietherapy with non-radioactive preparation), *British J. of Radiology, 40:*184-186, 1967.
2. Pierquin, B.: "Dosimetry: The Relational System." Proceedings of a Conference in New York City. May 6—8, 1971. *Afterloading in Radiotherapy:* 204-227. U.S. Department of Health, Education and Welfare. Bureau of Radiological Health. Rockville, Maryland, 1971.
3. Pierquin, B., and Fayos, J.V.: Dosimetry by tomography in interstitial curietherapy: point technique. *American J. of Roentegenology, 87:*585-592, 1962.

4. Pierquin B., Dutreix, A., Wambersie, A., Chassagne, D., and Stella, J.: La dosimétrie provisionnele en endocuriethérapie (dispositif radifere en un plan: étude sur ordinateur), *J. de Radiologie, 50:*377-383, 1969.

5. Pierquin, B.: A propos de la dose optima dans les cancers malphigiens; le concept des 2 volumes — cibles, *J. de Radiologie, 40:*545-547, 1959.

6. Wambersie, A., Dutreix, A., Pierquin, B., et Dardenne, J.C.: *Etude par ordinateur dans la répartition des doses autour de lignes radioactives paralléles, application dans un plan, Actes du Collogue sur l'utilisation des ordinateurs en radiologie,* to be published by S. Karger edit.

7. Wambersie, A., Dutreix, A., Pierquin, B., et Dardenne, J.C.: Dosimétrie provisionnelle en, thérapie intérstitelle au moyen de fils d' Iridium 192 (Le systeme de Paris). Applications dans un plan. Journal bèlge de Radiologie., *55:*197-206, 1972.

8. Paine, Ch., Pierquin, B., Dutreix, A., et Chassagne, D.: Dosimétrie des épingles d'Iridium 192 (étude théorique par ordinateur), *Annales de Radiologie, 12:*549-555, 1969.

9. Cameron, J. R., Suntharalingam, N., and Kenney, G. N.,: *Thermo-luminescent Dosimetry,* Milwaukee and London, 1968, Madison edit.

10. Devois, A., Decker, R., et Siboulet: La dosimétrie en curiethérapie: présentation d'un appareil de reproduction spatiale des punctures, *J. de Radiologie, 39:*333-335, 1958.

11. Mussell, L. E.: The rapid reconstruction of radium implants: a new technique *British J. of Radiology, 29:*402-407. 1956.

12. Jacob, P., Abbatucci, J., et Martinet, J. P.: Téchnique de re pérage et de dosimétrie en curiethérapie, *J. de Radiologie, 40:*74-76, 1959.

13. Egan, R., and Johnson, G.C.: Multisection transverse tomography in radium implant calculations, *Radiology, 74:*407, 1960.

14. Schlienger, M., Rosenwald, J. C., Miclutia, M., Quint, R., et Pierquin, B.: Le controle dosimétrique en brachycuriethérapie (Iridium 192) par les isodoses "escargot", *Acta Radiologica,9:*282-288, 1970.

15. Shalek, R. J. and Stovall, M. A.: Calculation of isodose distributions in interstitial implantations by computer, *Radiology, 76:*119-120, 1961.

16. Dutreix, A.: Utilisation d'un ordinateur pour la dosimétrie en curie-thérapie, *Annales de physique biologique et médicale, 2:*139-146, 1967.

17. Rosenwald, J. C., Dutreix, A., Chassagne, D., et Pierquin, B: Calcul sur ordinateur de la distribution réélle des doses autour d'une implantation intérstitielle de boucles ou épingles d'Iridium 192. *J., de Radiologie d'éléctrologie et de médecine nucléaire, 54:*47-50, 1973.

Chapter VI

THE ORGANIZATION OF A DEPARTMENT OF BRACHYTHERAPY

A section of brachytherapy is normally included in a department of radiation therapy equipped with all necessary technical and hospital facilities for treating patients with ionizing radiations. We will review the appropriate locales and technicalities of brachytherapy, problems of protection and the functional aspects for a typical department of radiation therapy.

I. THE DEPARTMENT OF BRACHYTHERAPY

A department of brachytherapy consists of a suite of three rooms; a room for the storage and preparation of radioactive material, a hot lab, and an application room.

A. Storage and Preparation Room

This room can be rather small (4 x 2.5 meters) and should contain:

—a storage container for Iridium 192

—two or three portable containers for Iridium 192

—at least two storage containers for Cesium 137

—a work table for the preparation of radioactive materials

—a sink equipped with running water

—a linear probe for checking the activity of Iridium 192 and Cesium 137 sources

—a storage and preparation table for Phosphorus 32, Strontium 90 and Yttrium 90 applicators.

B. The Iridium 192 Storage Container

The container is composed of a horizontal, armored and insulated core forming a storage keg which revolves within two fixed armored and insulated walls (Figure 39).*

This keg contains 456 vertical channels which receive removable stainless steel sleeves. These sleeves of varying lengths contain the radioactive sources (Figure 40).

*Establishment Lemer, Nantes (France).

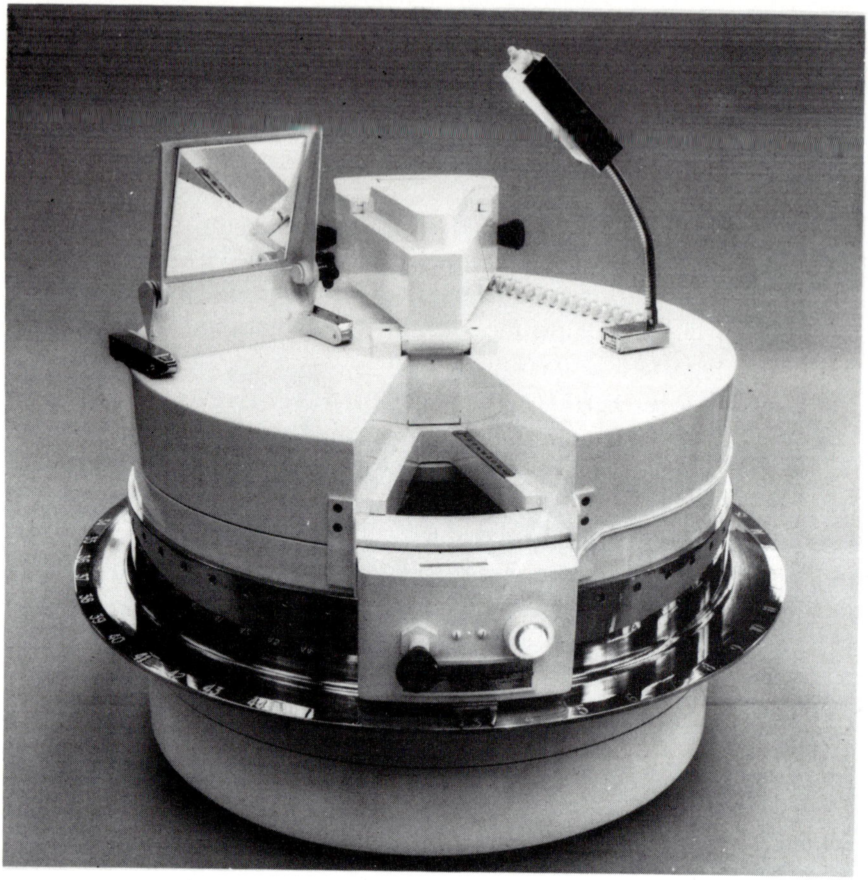

Figure 39. The shielded storage container for 1^{192} wire sources.

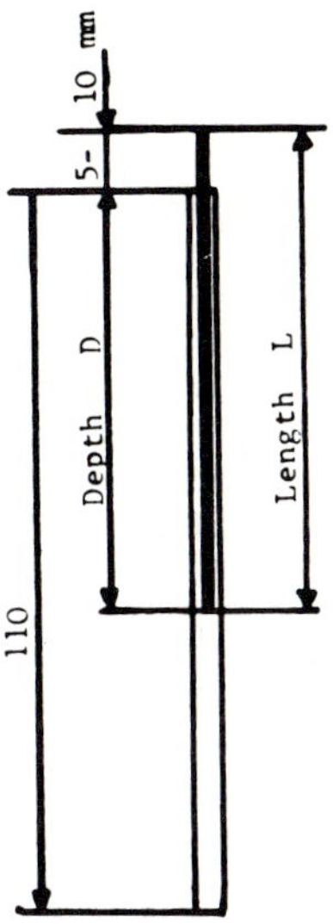

Type	Depth D	Length of Wire L
1	15	20 - 25
2	20	25 - 30
3	25	30 - 35
4	30	35 - 40
5	35	40 - 45
6	40	45 - 50
7	45	50 - 55
8	50	55 - 60
9	55	60 - 65
10	60	65 - 70
11	65	70 - 75
12	70	75 - 80
13	75	80 - 85
14	80	85 - 90
15	85	90 - 95
16	90	95 - 100
17	95	100 - 105
18	100	105 - 110
19	105	110 - 115

Figure 40. Cross sectional diagram and portion of the 1^{192} stock book showing the position and type of sources in the number coded channels. Pin heads extend 5 — 10 mm above the pig allowing rapid handling.

A door opening on top gives access to the container. This door can be locked and there is a light which functions when it is unlocked (Figure 41).

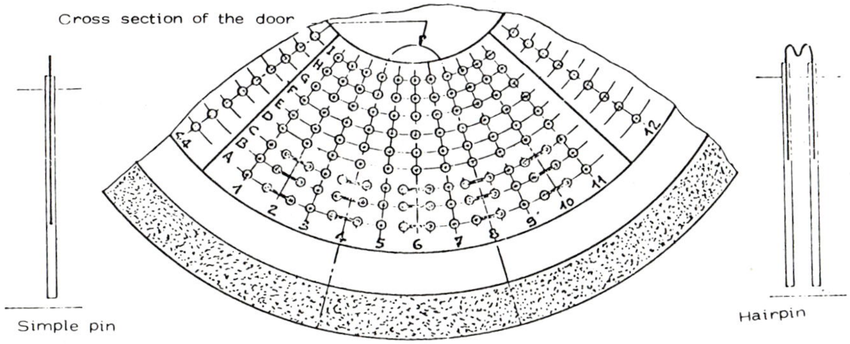

Figure 41. Top view through open door of 1^{192} storage container.

An adjustable mirror gives a full view of the elements within the container.

The container is supported on soft wheels and may be kept either on an existing countertop or on a special accessory table. The total weight of the container is about 300 Kilos.

C. The Linear Activimeter

Determination of the linear activity (activity per cm of radioactive length) is necessary for the sources used in photon therapy, namely, Iridium 192 or Cesium 137. The use of this apparatus is justified for the following reasons:

A. The radiotherapist has the moral and legal responsibility for the treatment and should, therefore, be able to personally verify the activity of the material used. Additionally, he often cuts portions of the wire in order to adapt the material to the particular conditions of the treatment which may alter the linear activity. Finally, several wires or Cesium seeds of different linear activities may be available simultaneously, inviting the possibility of confusion.

B. These instruments measure the total activity at the time of utilization by means of a simple reading. They eliminate any possible confusion and the need for calculations of decay that the material has sustained. Their operation is rather simple, making use of an ionization chamber (Figure 42).

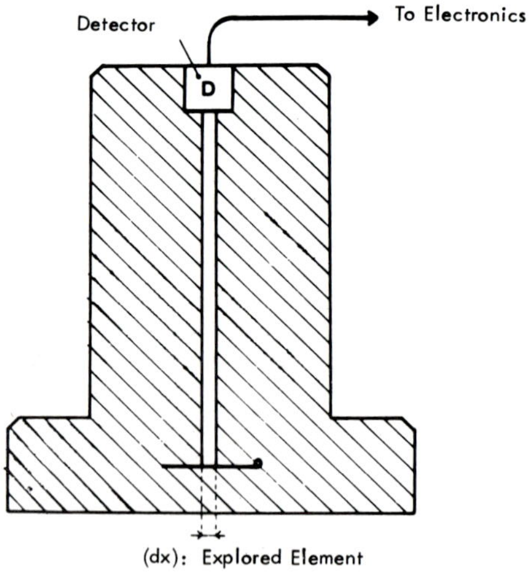

Figure 42. Diagram of the Linear Activimeter.

This very precise method presents certain inconveniences in brachytherapy, however:

a. Although measuring the length of straight wires is relatively easy, wire pins that have already been previously used in several applications and have been bent are more difficult to measure. Resultant inaccuracies are projected in the value of the linear activity.

For example, an error of 1mm in the length of a 3 cm wire will result in an error of more than 3% in the linear activity.*

b. These complementary measurements of the length result in increasing the dose received by the operator.

c. Finally, certain linear activimeters are too small to accurately measure long sources without first modifying the initial configuration of these elements. For example, wires 14 cm long or certain long pins.

C. It is, therefore, necessary to directly measure the linear activity of these materials and it is also of use in verifying their homogeneity, which can also be determined using such an apparatus.

We have commissioned the manufacture of equipment which permits us to accomplish these measurements, namely, the linear electrometer (Figure 43).

II. APPLICATION ROOM

This is a large room measuring at least 5 x 8 meters, containing a surgical table, and a brachytherapy installation which permits the sitting and horizontal positioning of patients. This room is equipped as an operating room, allowing work under sterile conditions and with the necessary comforts, such as tiled surfaces, operating room lights, sinks with foot control, linens and instrument boxes for general surgery, general anesthesia and for resuscitation (Figure 44).

For the sitting position, there is a chair with an adjustable head holder and a televised fluoroscopy unit that can be fixed in any desired position. The setup for horizontal positioning deserves special description. We will describe briefly the installation in one of our departments of brachytherapy.

*Establishment Lascaux — Limoges (France).

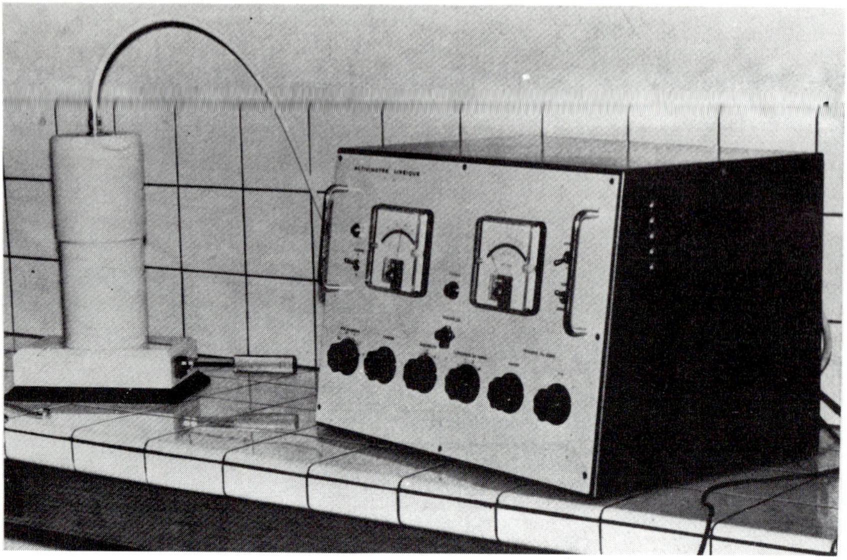

Figure 43. The linear electrometer.

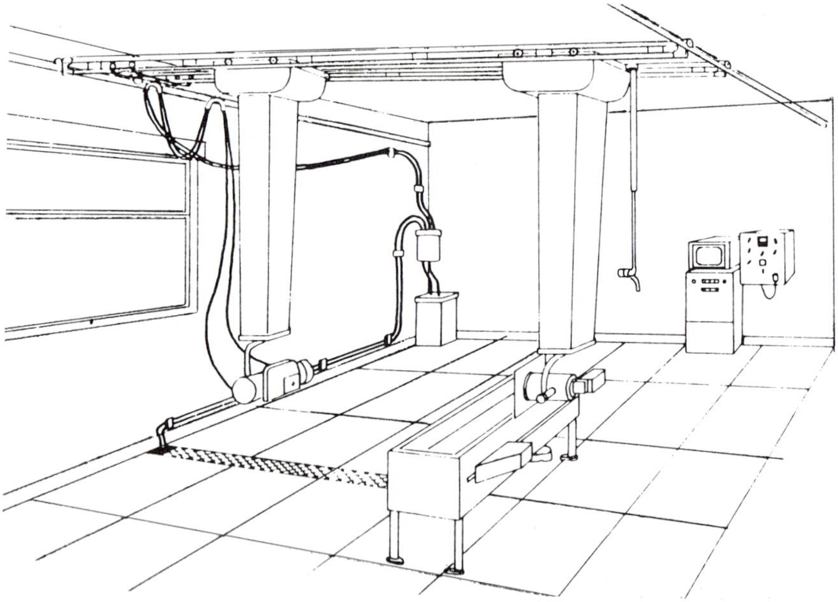

Figure 44. Diagram of the application room in a typical department of brachytherapy. The television sets are on mobile carts.

It consists of a fixed table, an x-ray unit with two tubes, an image amplification screen and several television sets. The table is mounted on a fixed frame with four legs; its top is movable allowing positioning of the head and the lithotomy position. On either side, one can attach trays. The two x-ray tubes are placed in an orthogonal position; the vertical one mounted on a ceiling bridge on a telescopic arm. Each of the x-ray tubes can be placed in coincidence on the normal radius with an image amplifier. The amplifier can also be oriented in a vertical or horizontal position, and is also attached to the moving bridge by a telescopic arm. A television camera is connected to the optical system of the amplifier. The brachytherapist can thus follow radioscopically, on the television screens, the different phases of the implantation. After the application, marker films can be taken with frontal and lateral views, and the films are developed in the immediate vicinity. When computer dosimetry is contemplated, a special cassette holder with automatic centering is used. This setup can also be used for patients in the sitting position.

III.. THE HOT LAB

This is a small room, approximately 3 x 4 meters, where deliveries of radioactive materials can be received and for disposing of radioactive wastes. A "well chamber" is desirable for measuring the activity of any shipments.

For disposing of wastes, especially Iridium 192 wires or pins, a "cemetery" safe, made of concrete, is useful. These are returned to the manufacturer every 6 to 12 months after being checked by the radiation protection officer.

IV. PROTECTION

Radiation protection is the major problem in the organization of a department of brachytherapy. In teletherapy, the radiation source is sealed within a well protected apparatus which is permanently installed in a perfectly protected room. It is activated from a control area outside of the treatment room, under conditions of protection which are nearly absolute. In endo- and plesiotherapy, protection can only be relative, for in all work areas, some irradiation of the personnel is inevitable. A brachytherapist should be aware of protection requirements, detect the "hot areas" of his department where the danger to the personnel is highest, and work in close collaboration with the Department of Radiation Physics in order to reduce or eliminate the causes of unnecessary irradiation.

Legislation concerning the protection of the personnel is now well established by the International Commission of Protection Against Radiations, whose recommendations adopted in 1954 and in 1958, have become part of the law[4,5]. Permissible doses are measured in rem; one rem corresponding to the risk sustained by the human organism that receives a dose of 1 rad of x rays or gamma rays. The maximum permissible dose is 5 rems per year, that is 0.1 rem per week, corresponding to a dose of 2.5 millirem per hour for a 40 hour work week. These figures represent averages allowing possible fluctuations, provided the maximum accumulated dose does not exceed 3 rems in 13 consecutive weeks. However, the law allows larger doses when only part of the body is irradiated. In brachythereapy, one may receive a dose of 20 rems in 13 weeks, or 1.5 rem per week to the hands.

The "hot areas" in the department of brachytherapy should be well known and posted.

In the storage areas, conditions of protection are fairly uniform and stable. The radioactive material is locked in containers, the hot areas not exceeding 2.5 mR per hour on the surface of the containers. Although this risk is not critical, it is, no less real in time. The entire room is, in effect, submitted to a feeble continuous irradiation. It is, therefore, advisable to avoid remaining in this room for prolonged periods of time, and to use it only for the transit of the radioactive material.

In the preparation area, hot areas should be checked for with vigilance, especially on the work tables. A lead shield 3 cm thick should adequately protect the operator against whole body irradiation [6]. The protection of the hands, which are inevitably closer to the radioactive sources, is considered on a different basis. The brachytherapist should coordinate all his body movements and learn well how to use long forceps, and to remove all excess radioactive sources from the work area. In the preparation room, his exemplary performance is essential for benefit of trainees.

In the application room, no complete protection can be interposed between the operator and the patient during the application of the radioactive material. This is precisely why afterloading techniques have developed to the utmost, to avoid any irradiation during the placement of the guide systems. During the introduction and substitution of the radioactive material, adequate protection can be offered by lead screens, with the operator remaining at a distance from the patient, and using long forceps or remote controls. Protection with lead screens that do not exceed 2 to 3 cm in thickness is not cumbersome. We especially recommend the use of movable lead screens 2 cm thick (Figure 45).

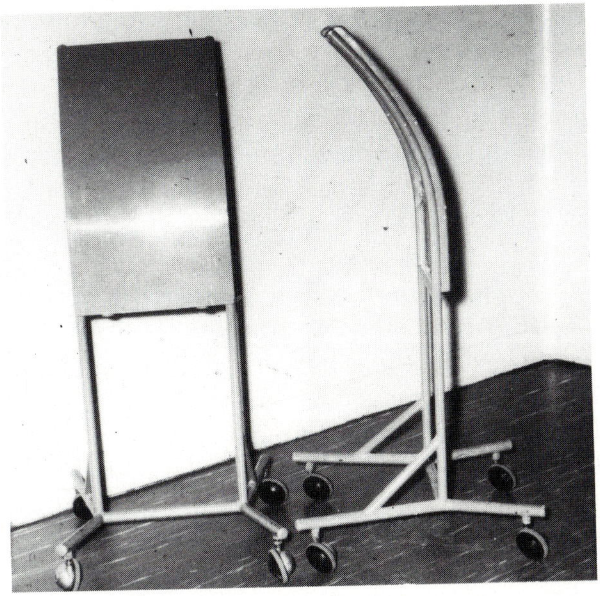

Figure 45. Mobile lead screens provide effective protective barriers in a brachytherapy department.

Some of these screens are straight, 30 cm wide and 120 cm high, while others are curved to allow the operator to lean over the patient. They move very easily on coasters, and can be put into position in a few seconds around the operating area to protect the physician and his assistants. Three straight panels and three curved panels are needed in the usual application room [6].

A container for Iridium 192 sources can also be connected to these movable screens. Ordinarily they do not weigh more than 15 kilos and offer satisfactory protection (Figure 8).

One should insist on the practical importance of the mobile protection, which, for the low energy of Iridium 192, assures at any time and in any area of the department of brachytherapy an immediate and efficient protection.

In the patients room, the patients constitute foci of radiations against which the protection of the personnel administering direct care such as dressings, injections, etc. is more difficult. The nurse should, therefore, expedite her work, postponing any conversation or any act not requiring her presence near the patient. She should maintain a minimum distance of 1.5 meters from the bed, and remain behind lead screens whenever possible. As to the family, visits should be limited to a few minutes, with absolute restrictions for children or pregnant women. In gynecology, the development and the use of remote afterloaders has simplified protection problems.

III. THE FUNCTIONING OF A DEPARTMENT OF BRACHYTHERAPY

This section concerns the internal organization of a department and its relationship with nuclear centers.

Internal functioning of a department is a delicate matter since it must take into account unforeseeable fluctuations in the work schedule, the variations in radioactivity of different batches of the same source material, and predictable and unpredictable differences in the geometry of the radioactive setup for each anatomic location and in each individual case. The result is that the time of application and the duration of irradiation varies from week to week, and from patient to patient.

For practical purposes, in most cases of endotherapy or plesiotherapy the application time is short, varying from a few minutes to a few hours, for benign cutaneous lesions, or relatively long, that is about 4 to 6 days, for malignant lesions. Hospitalization during long applications is, therefore, of the order of one week. Practically, however, the admission and discharge of patients can be carried out only on a day-to-day basis because of the important unforeseeable fluctuations mentioned. Regularization of the program of daily work is possible by performing technically major applications which require general anesthesia and a radiosurgical association, on two or three pre-established days of the week. The simpler short applications can be done at any time during a working day.

One should remember that removal of the radioactive material may be required at any hour requiring a call system for physicians and technicians, including Sundays and holidays.

The relationship with the supplying nuclear center should develop beyond the administrative level. Brachytherapists should establish a personal relationship with the responsible authorities of the Department of Radioactive Elements of their nuclear center, resulting in a fruitful collaboration in research as well as routine work.

Routinely, a practical method should be established to request regular orders, and radioactive materials should be chosen which are used in as large a number of radiation centers as possible. It is, in fact, always difficult for a nuclear center to guarantee the same specific activity for the same radioactive materials from one order to the next, because unforeseeable variations in the flux of neutrons during the course of activation is very common. This factor is even more pronounced if the material to be radioactivated is not placed in the same channel of irradiation in the atomic pile, since the flux of radiations varies greatly from one location to another within the pile. Additionally, the presence of other materials placed next to the one ordered can act as a barrier to neutrons and diminish the desired level of radioactivity. Two or three fold variations are sometimes encountered. To minimize these difficulties, one ought to order any given radioactive material from a single nuclear center so that the producer reserves an identical position within the pile giving the order preferential treatment during each activation cycle.

This is why we have established, at the Nuclear Center of Saclay, France, an Iridium 192 bank that receives orders from about 30 users, guaranteeing the immediate delivery (within 48 hours) of certain types of radioactive materials with a radioactivity varying by not more than 5% between shipments. In order to have an effective bank of this type, a minimum of 12 users is necessary (Figure 46)[7].

WIRES		PINS			
Wire of 0.3 mm. (1) in diameter	Wire of 0.5 mm. in diameter	Simple Pins		Hairpin	
		L = 3 cm.	L = 5 cm.	L = 3 cm.	L = 5 cm.
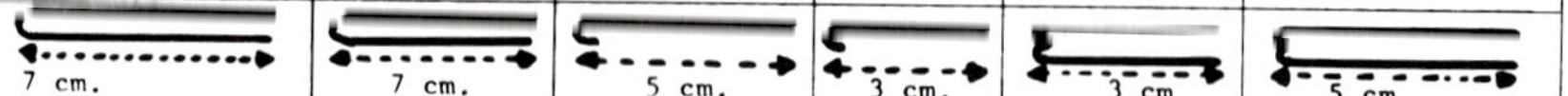					
7 cm. 14 cm.	7 cm. 14 cm.	5 cm. 3 cm.	3 cm. 5 cm.	3 cm. 3 cm.	5 cm. 5 cm.

(1) This wire is available for a total length of 14 cm. It is bent in 2 to fit in the container the height of which does not exceed 7 cm.

Figure 46. The Iridium 192 bank. Table of the typical sizes and types of Iridium 192 wire sources available to users of the bank.

REFERENCES

1. Piérquin, B: Le dévelopement de la radiothérapie, *La Presse Médicale, 75:*2577-2579, 1967.
2. Bernard, M., et Dutirex, A.: Dispositif de mesure de 1 ăctivimètre linéique, *J. de Radiologie, 49:*534-537, 1968.
3. Piérquin, B., et Chassagne, D.: L iridium 192 et le Césium 137 dans les pérspéctives du recent décret sur la protéction contre les radiations ionisantes, *J. de Radiologie, 49:*533-534, 1968.
4. Récommendations de la Commission Intérnationale de la Protéction contre les Radiations ionisantes — 1° Décembre, 1954, *J. de Radiologie, 36;* Supplément N° 10 bis, 1955.
5. *Récommendations de la Commission Intérnational de la Protéction contre les Radiations ionisantes - Séptembre, 1958,* Londres, 1959, Pergamon Press.
6. Pierquin, B.: Colloque sur la protéction en curiethérapie (sources Scéllés), *J. de Radiologie, 48:*38-42, 1967.
7. Piérquin, B.: Journée d'Information sur 1'Iridium 192, *Annales de Radiologie, 8:*593-594, 1965.

Chapter VII

CLINICAL APPLICATIONS

We will limit our discussion in each case to the techniques which appear advisable to us. For each location, the presentation will be according to the following format:

a. A clinical anatomical review with a brief description of the anatomic conditions and the clinical and histopathological characteristics of neoplasms arising in that site.

b. A description of the recommended technique.

c. A brief discussion of the results of treatment.

UPPER AERODIGESTIVE PASSAGES

The indications for endotherapy or plesiotherapy in these regions are numerous and are often the treatment of choice. Carcinomas arising in these areas are, in fact, remarkably well treated by brachytherapy, due to their easy accessibility and because they are often detected at an early stage of development.

We will successively discuss the indications for brachytherapy in the treatment of lesions of the nasopharynx, the nasal fossa, the sinuses, the oropharynx, the oral cavity and the hypopharynx. Additionally, we will review the use of brachytherapy in the management of metastatic disease in cervical lymph nodes.

The upper air passages are essentially natural cavities consisting of the maxillary and ethmoid sinuses, the nasal fossae and the nasopharynx. They are relatively inaccessible to instrumentation, and in view of this difficulty, the use of brachytherapy in these regions is by surface applicators only. The target volume of this method may not extend beyond a depth of 10-12 mm. from the surface of the mucous membranes; therefore, the technique should not be used for infiltrating tumors, except when the bulk of the tumor has been surgically removed, leaving only a thin layer of residual tumor. This combined approach is possible in tumors of the maxillary antrum and ethmoid sinuses. In the nasopharynx, plesiotherapy should be used only for the treatment of superficial and minimally infiltrating lesions.

Although most of these lesions are epidermoid carcinomas, the indications for plesiotherapy of the nasal fossa are mainly for benign familial hereditary hemangiomas (Rendu-Osler disease), especially by the plastic tube technique. We have eliminated from this book any recommendation for plesiotherapy of adenoids of the nasopharynx. The use of the Crowe applicator and other gamma emitters for this purpose should be abandoned because of the radiation hazard to the patient. In view of the inflammatory character of these lesions, they can be treated quite adequately with other non-radiotherapeutic modalities.

Nasopharynx

a. Clinical Anatomical Review — The nasopharynx is a cavity lying between the nasal fossa and the pharynx. Its accessibility to instrumentation is very difficult, and one can only approach it indirectly by using radioactive applicators. For epidermoid carcinomas, including lymphoepitheliomas, one can deliver a supplementary boost dose with plesiotherapy following the administration of a basic dose with teletherapy, when the tumor is limited to the mucous membranes of the roof, the lateral or posterior walls of the nasopharynx.

b. Recommended Technique — We recommend a technique of plesiotherapy by plastic tubes fixed on a mold applicator (patient supine, combination of local and basal anesthesia).

The technique consists of placing two to four radioactive sources of Iridium 192 wires in plastic tubes sagittally oriented within the nasopharynx. These tubes are immobilized on a polyvinyl applicator constructed from a mold of the nasopharynx.[2,3]

Preparation of the Patient

The patient is prepared with basal anesthesia, maintaining the pharyngeal reflexes and a relative muscular tonicity. Then the mucous membranes are locally anesthetized through the nasal fossa and the oral cavity with a spray of 10% Xylocaine. Thus the brachytherapist can work in the oral cavity, the nasal fossa and the nasopharynx without triggering the gag reflex or pain, and without intubating the patient.

Preparation of the Applicator

a. Impression of the nasopharynx — one starts by introducing a #12 rubber catheter into each nostril. The buccal end of each rubber catheter is then connected to a thread to which a dummy applicator is attached. This applicator is much smaller than the normal nasopharynx, and is covered with a quick drying plastic paste. By pulling on the nasal catheters, this dummy applicator covered with the paste is brought through the oral cavity, passes behind the soft palate to come in contact with the walls of the nasopharynx, allowing the paste to over flow slightly towards the posterior choanes of the nasal fossa. The paste hardens in two to three minutes; but remains quite elastic and is easily removable from the nasopharynx. A very accurate impression is thus obtained, outlining the details of the lesion without the necessity of applying any deforming pressure on the mucosa of the nasopharynx. If this model appears defective, one repeats the procedure adding more paste to the defective parts of the mold.

The patient is kept under basal anesthesia while the technician constructs the plastic applicator.

b. Construction of the plastic applicator: A plaster of Paris mold is first made from which the plastic applicator is prepared using a polyvinyl paste. The contours of this plastic applicator are smoothed with a grinder. A double nylon thread is attached to its lower posterior aspect to be used during its later extraction. At the upper and anterior aspect, two small rubber strips are attached at the level of the small projections which extend into each choane, which will be used to maintain the radioactive setup in position by pulling them gently through the nostrils [19].

c. Placement of the nylon guide tubes on the plastic applicator: The brachytherapist then defines the desired position of each radioactive source, in relationship to the location and the extent of the tumor, which as stated, has usually left its imprint on the impression. The boundaries of the tumor are first drawn on the surface of the applicator and the desired position of each radioactive source is marked with a sagittal line. The roof and the posterior surface of the nasopharynx form, in effect, one curved surface in the sagittal plane. The space between the sources varies between 10 and 12 mm. In an average size nasopharynx, one can usually place two sources on one lateral wall, three sources on two walls, for example, the roof and one lateral wall, or four sources on three walls.

Grooves are made corresponding to the lines drawn on the applicator, to cradle the outer plastic guide tubes with sealed ends. These are about 20 cm long and are glued in place with more polyvinyl paste.

Before inserting the applicator, it is important to check the setup using dummy sources. The exact length of the Iridium 192 wire to be loaded into each tube is then carefully measured and the different tubes are identified by cutting them at slightly different lengths. This preparation requires a total of about 1 to 2 hours (Figure 47).

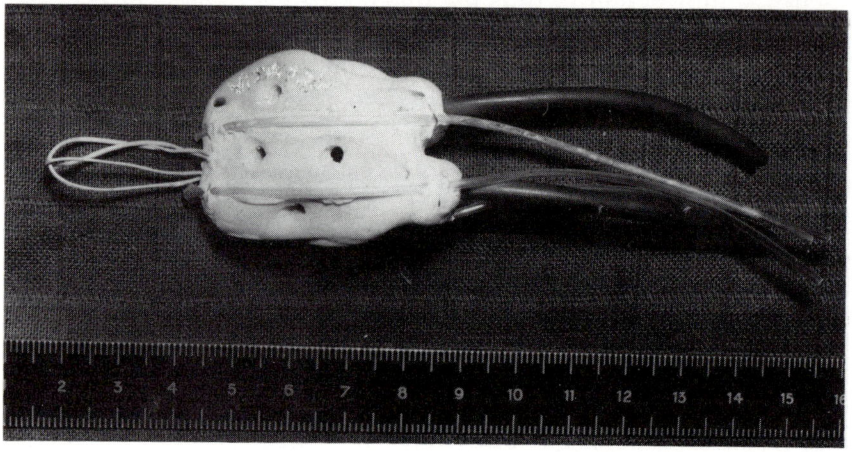

Figure 47. Cancer of the nasopharynx. Completed plastic applicator.

Insertion of the Applicator

Any mucous is carefully suctioned first, and an antibiotic powder is applied on the mucous membranes of the nasopharynx.

The rubber nasal catheters used initially, are reinserted avoiding any crossover in the nasopharynx.

The plastic applicator is then placed, "upside down," on the patient's chest. The rubber strips and outer plastic tubes are then introduced into the distal end of the corresponding nasal catheter for a length of about 2 to 3 cm and a ligature is placed around the latter and tied firmly.

While elevating the soft palate with a retractor, the two nasal catheters are pulled simultaneously from the nasal end. The plastic applicator thus penetrates the oral cavity, slides behind the soft palate and falls naturally into place to exactly fit the nasopharynx.

The rubber strips and the plastic tubes are then disengaged from the nasal catheters and the strips are tied together in front of the nasal septum, with light traction, leaving only the free ends of the nylon tubes projecting in air. Immobilization buttons are then slid over each plastic tube to the level of the nasal orifices. The setup is now ready to receive the radioactive material, following a final check and after establishing the dosimetry (Figure 48).

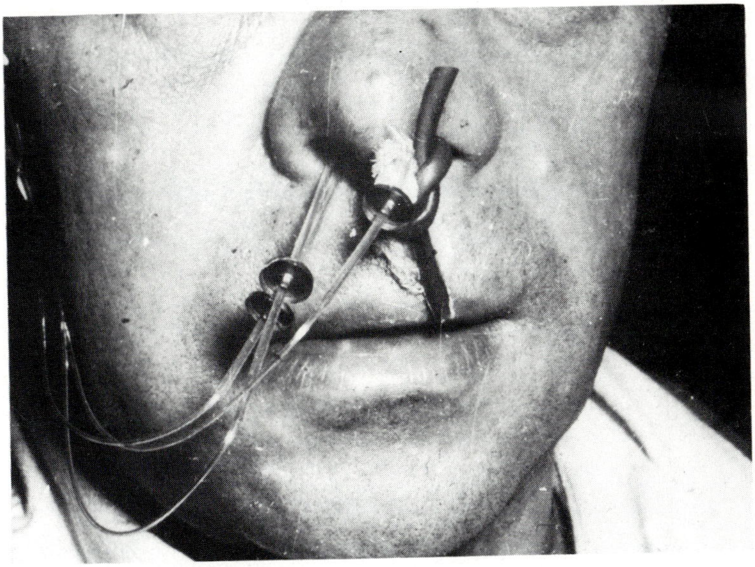

Figure 48. Cancer of the nasopharynx. The final position of the nasopharyngeal applicator.

Dosimetry

Lead wires of the desired length are introduced into each nylon tube. With fluoroscopy, their exact pre-established position and lengths are verified. At this time, marker films (Figure 49 (a, b)) and a unidirectional tomogram, perpendicular to the sagittal direction of the tubes is made (Figure 49 c). On a sketch made from this tomogram, the spatial dosimetry at the level of the mucous membranes and the bony structures of the nasopharynx is established. In general, a significant thickness of tissue of up to 10

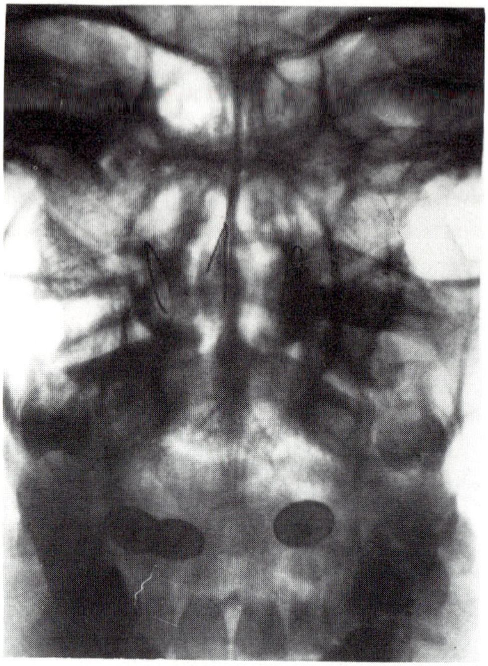

Figure 49. Cancer of the nasopharynx. Marker films and tomogram obtained with dummy sources in applicator.
a. Frontal view

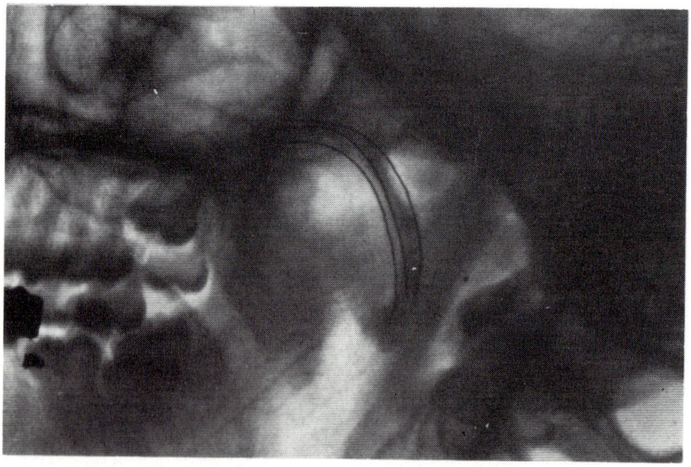

Figure 49. b. Lateral view

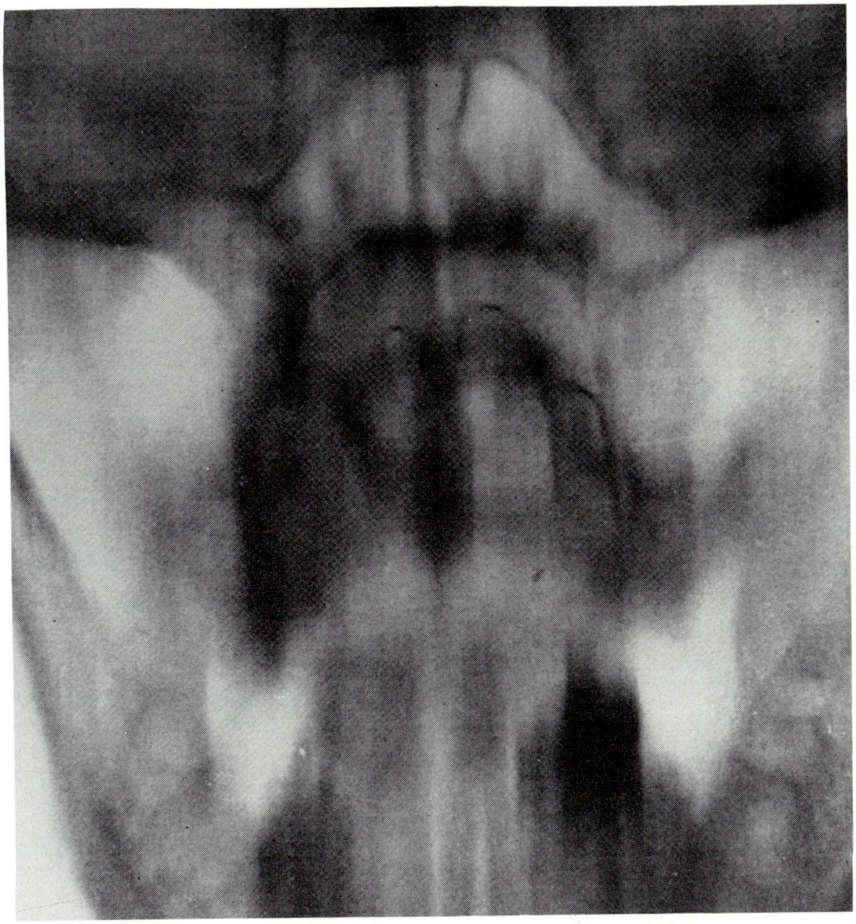

Figure 49. c. Frontal tomogram

mm is noted between the mucous membrane of the roof or posterior wall of the nasopharynx and the adjacent bones.

Without great risk to the surrounding bony structures, a total dose of the order of 4000 rads, when combined with teletherapy, and 7000 rads when plesiotherapy alone is used can be achieved without difficulty (Figure 49 d). These doses are calculated at a depth of 0.5 to 1 cm depth depending upon the anatomy.

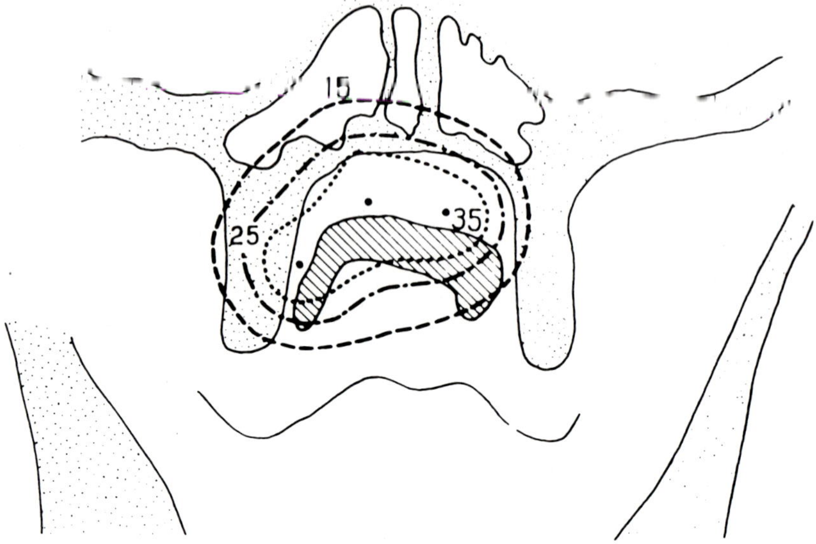

Figure 49. d. Dosimetry derived from the tomogram
Reference isodose = isodose 25 rad/hr.
Required tumor dose = 4000 rad (boost following teletherapy)
Activity of I^{192} wires = 1.3 m Ci/cm
Duration of application = $\frac{4000}{25 \times 1.3}$ = 123 hrs.

Insertion of the Iridium 192 Wires

After identifying each outer tube carefully, the Iridium 192 wires are loaded into small inner tubes and inserted into the appropriate larger tube. They are immobilized by crushing buttons onto the tubes.

Monitoring During the Course of the Application

During the few days of the application, the patient is maintained with a medical regimen of antibiotics, analgesics and tranquilizers, and a liquid or semi-liquid diet. This custom-made applicator generally remains well positioned and does not interfere with sleeping.

It is important to aspirate the nasal discharge that may accumulate at the nares several times during the day.

Extraction of the Material

a. The inner tubes containing the Iridium 192 wires are removed first.

b. The applicator is then easily removed by cutting the rubber strips in front of the nasal septum, removing the immobilization buttons and by then pulling on the nylon threads attached to the applicator through the oral cavity. This will result in the rapid extraction of the applicator from behind the soft palate.

c. *Therapeutic Results:* Since 1962, we have treated 62 patients with this technique. All cases were epidermoid carcinomas (T-1 and T-2), irradiated initially with telecobalt therapy (4500 rads), followed by plesiotherapy adding an additional dose of 4000 rads, for a total dose of 8500 rads. Fifteen of 24 patients (62%) remained well without evidence of local recurrence at three years. There was no instance of radionecrosis in these patients[40]. We especially recommend consideration of this technique for treating small localized recurrences.

Nasal Fossa

a. *Clinical Anatomical Review* — we will consider only the treatment of diffuse mucosal hemangiomas or Rendu-Osler disease. Malignant tumors are, in fact, very rare in the nasal fossa and will be reviewed with malignant tumors of the nose.

The nasal fossae are in the form of narrow crevices separated by a cartilagenous septum, the usual deformity of which yields a somewhat larger fossa on one side. Their walls form a right angle triangle with the right angle situated in the lower and posterior corner where the choanes join the floor of the nasal fossa, and with the long side following the dorsum of the nose, to become more horizontal superiorly at the level of the cribriform plate. These crevices are wide at the level of the floor and become gradually more narrow towards the superior margin in view of the presence of the inferior, middle and superior turbinates.

In cases of diffuse hemangiomas extending over the entire mucosal surface of the nasal fossae, a delicate problem is created in establishing a uniform distribution of dose.

b. *Recommended Technique* — We recommend the plastic tube technique (local anesthesia, sitting position).

Three radioactive sources should adequately irradiate the entire mucosal surface of each fossa. The lower source should be in contact with or at a short distance from the floor, the middle source lies between the lower and middle turbinates and the upper source follows the dorsum of the nose to lie near the inferior surface of the cribriform plate. To avoid hot spots around the nasal opening where the three sources diverge, the length of the middle source is reduced, and its distal portion lies between the inferior and middle turbinates.

c. Therapeutic Results — Since 1960, we have treated 44 patients with this technique. A satisfactory result has been achieved in 60% of the new cases treated. No radionecrosis has been observed in the new cases treated with Iridium 192.

Maxillary and Ethmoid Sinuses

a. Clinical Anatomical Review — Two groups of malignant tumors of the maxillary sinuses can be identified grossly; those arising from the infrastructure and those of the suprastructure. This distinction is only valid for lesions of moderate size (T_2 or T_3). Malignant tumors of the infrastructure are usually treated by surgical resection, alone. Plesiotherapy is used in these cases only if the lesions are found to be quite extensive at the time of surgery. Total surgical removal of malignant tumors of the suprastructure is exceedingly difficult. In these cases, plesiotherapy can be used advantageously to a certain extent.

b. Recommended Technique — We recommend a plastic applicator technique of plesiotherapy utilizing plastic tubes containing Iridium 192 wires (patient supine, basal anesthesia).
This application is performed postoperatively, usually one week after the surgical intervention into the maxillary or ethmoid sinuses. An oral prosthesis is used to support the mold when the infrastructure has been removed.

The optimum dose is variable in view of the different clinical and therapeutic indications. It is usually between 4000 and 7000 rads at a depth of 8-10 mm beyond the walls of the cavity.

c. Therapeutic Results — Since 1960, we have treated 27 patients with this technique. This small group of patients includes both new and recurrent cases and lesions of both infra- and suprastructure origin. With such small groups, no statistically significant therapeutic results can be stated. We observed, however, that of seven new patients followed for three years, only one local recurrence was seen.

REFERENCES

1. Flaisler, A., Markovits, P., et Pierquin, B.: Neuroléptanalgésie en radiologie, *J. de Radiologie, 47:*817-820, 1966.
2. Pierquin, B., Janvier, L., Chassagne, D., et Le cacheux, B.: Les appareils moules en curietherapie, *Actualités odonto — stomatologiques, 77:*61-75, 1967.
3. Chassagne, D., Janvier, L., Pierquin, B., et Flaisler, A.: La plésiocuriethérapie des cancers du cavum avec support — moule et Yridium 192, *Annales de Radiologie, 6:*719-726, 1963.
4. Pierquin, B., Cachin, Y., Chassagne, D., Le Fur, R., et Bigot, R.: Etude de 49 cas du cavum traités a l Institute Gustave Roussy de 1960 à 1965, *La Presse Médicale, 76:*1565-1566, 1968.
5. Pierquin, B., Koskas, Y., et Chassagne, D.: La plésiocuriethérapie endonasale de la maladie de Rendu — Osler par Iridium 192, *Annales d'Oto-Laryngologie, 86:*127-132, 1969.

Oropharynx

The relatively deep location of the oropharynx, its essential function in the first stage of deglutition and the gag reflex, make the instrumental access to the different structures of the oropharynx difficult. However, with the establishment of well defined techniques and especially with the use of artificial radioactive elements, endotherapy can be efficiently used in the oropharynx, whether treating the soft palate, the tonsillar regions, the base of the tongue or the posterior wall of the oropharynx.

There are three particular indications for endotherapy in the oropharynx:

1. For T_1 lesions following 5000 rads of external irradiation to give a "boost dose" of 3000 to 3500 rads.

2. When the patient has been previously treated with external irradiation for another primary. In such instances, brachytherapy alone, to a dose of 6500 to 7000 rads is given, accepting an increased risk of necrosis.

3. For well delimited localized recurrences.

Soft Palate

a. Clinical Anatomical Review — The soft palate is delimited superiorly and anteriorly by the hard palate and inferiorly by its own free margin including the uvula. Technically, we will describe the irradiation of malignant tumors limited to the soft palate excluding lesions of the palatotonsillar regions, which will be described later.

b. Recommended Technique — We recommend the guide gutter technique of endotherapy (local anesthesia, patient sitting). The technique of endotherapy with guide gutters for lesions of the oropharynx and for lesions elsewhere in general, includes a certain number of common details which will now be described.

The sitting position is indispensible in order to disengage the soft palate from the posterior wall of the oropharynx. The conscious state of the patient is also necessary to maintain a sufficient muscular tonicity in this thin muscle curtain. Experience has shown us that attempts at accomplishing endotherapy of the soft palate in a supine patient under general anesthesia is difficult and hazardous. The soft palate becomes very soft and flaccid, adhering to the posterior wall of the oropharynx and easily slips between the fingers of the therapist.

Preparation of the patient — the subject should be fasting under the influence of sedatives, and receive an injection of 0.5 mg of Atropine about 15 minutes before the procedure to control salivation. The subject sits in a chair equipped with head holder and an image intensifier, connected to television, is placed horizontally on either side of the patient's head. A few minutes before beginning the procedure, local anesthesia is achieved by giving the patient a lozenge of Tetracaine, followed by a spray of 10% Xylocaine to the entire oral and oropharyngeal mucosa.

The gag reflex is then tested in order to be assured that direct manipulation of the soft palate does not gag the patient.

The operator then injects about 10 to 15 cc of 1% Xylocaine with adrenalin into the soft palate. The point of injection is at the lateral border of the soft palate on the side of the implantation. The injection is made at this single point permitting the anesthesia to diffuse rapidly into the entire soft palate ballooning it. This ballooning of the soft palate plays an essential role in the insertion of the guides and must be utilized immediately.

Implantation of the Guide Gutters

Depending upon the extent of the tumor, two or three radioactive sources are usually inserted in a transverse direction from right to left or left to right, depending on which side the bulk of the lesion resides. The length of the tubes is about 3 to 4 cm. Their implantation will be practically impossible and very hazardous if the soft palate is not ballooned by the anesthetic agent. In fact, it becomes impossible to orient the guide in a transverse plane, since the soft palate lies deeply within the oral cavity. However, after the inflation with anesthetic, the anterior and posterior surface of the soft palate are separated from each other, making the implantation in an oblique direction posteromedially possible without risk of piercing its posterior surface. Within a few minutes, the anesthetic is absorbed and the branches of the guide gutters assume a normal transverse position.

Using the fluoroscope, the spacing and parallelism is carefully controlled by turning the patient's head to obtain frontal and lateral views. If a closed circuit television is focused on the image amplifier, control of the implantation of the guides and eventual corrections can be accomplished with even more ease by simply watching the television screen. When the guide is in good position, nylon sutures are placed through the mucosa passing under the transverse plaque of the guide. A large deep suture is preferable, leaving the two ends of each suture outside the oral cavity.

Insertion of the Radioactive Wires

Holding a nonserrated forceps in one hand, the operator applies firm traction on the plaque of the single or double guide gutter, in order to bring the latter into an adequate sagittal direction, and to be able to introduce the radioactive pin through the mouth. This maneuver is possible because of the great suppleness of the soft palate. With the other hand, the radioactive Iridium pin, held with nonserrated forceps, is introduced into the guides. The latter are simultaneously removed leaving the radioactive pins in place in the target volume. Usually, one hairpin 3 or 4 cm in length providing two radioactive lines is sufficient to encompass a moderately large lesion of the soft palate. If the tumor covers the entire soft palate, three lines are necessary, a hairpin plus a single pin (Figure 50a).

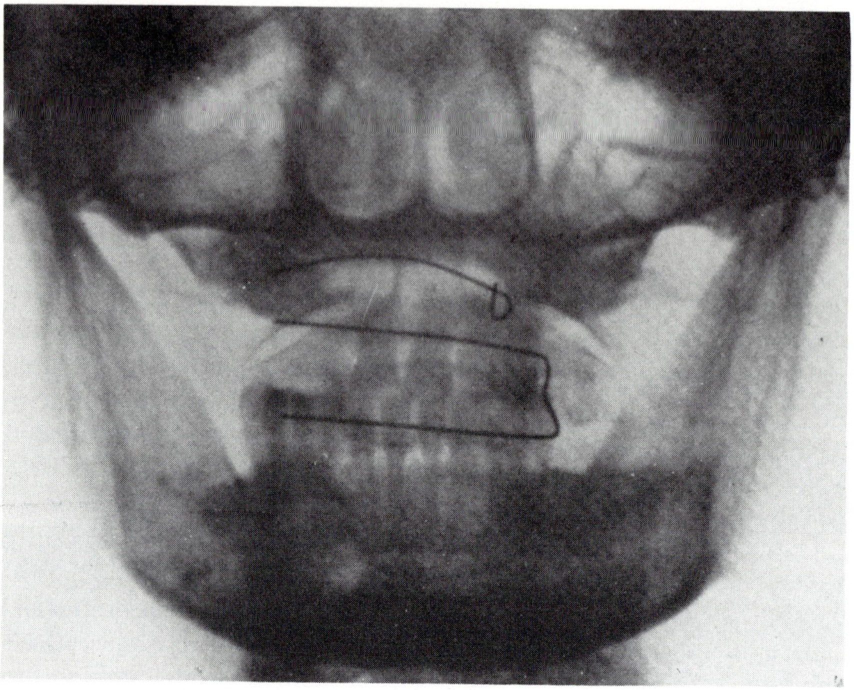

Figure 50. Carcinoma of the soft palate.
a. Implant consists of 3 radioactive lines, 1 hairpin and 1 single pin. Frontal view.

If the tumor extends to the inferior border of the soft palate or the uvula, one can treat it without difficulty by using a hairpin source, leaving part of its inferior branch free in air at the margin of the palate. Extra sutures will be necessary to hold it in this position.

The nylon sutures are then tied around the heads of the radioactive material and cut rather short.

With a little experience, this application can be accomplished in about 10 minutes. The radioactive exposure time does not usually exceed 2 or 3 minutes for the therapist.

As soon as the application is completed, frontal and lateral films are taken in order to check the position of the radioactive material (Figure 50 (a, b)). With the help of these marker films, the orientation of the sagittal tomography plane for dosimetry by points is established (Figure 50c).

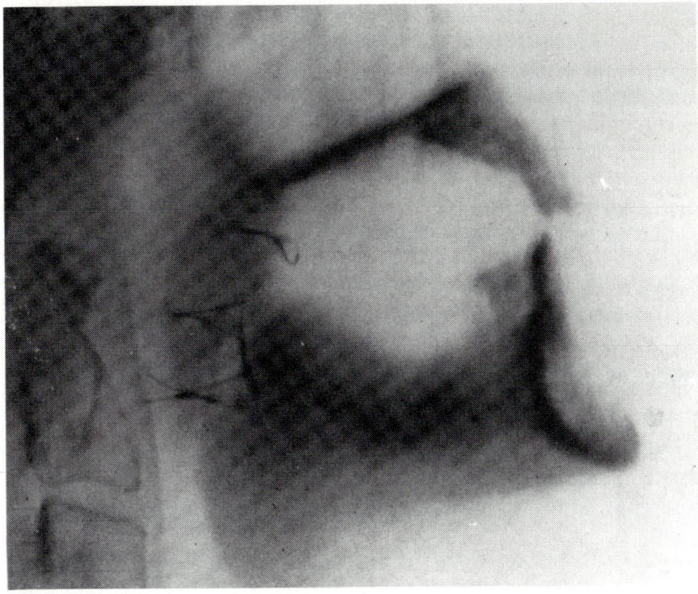

Figure 50.
b. Carcinoma of the soft palate. Tomogram in mid-sagittal plane.

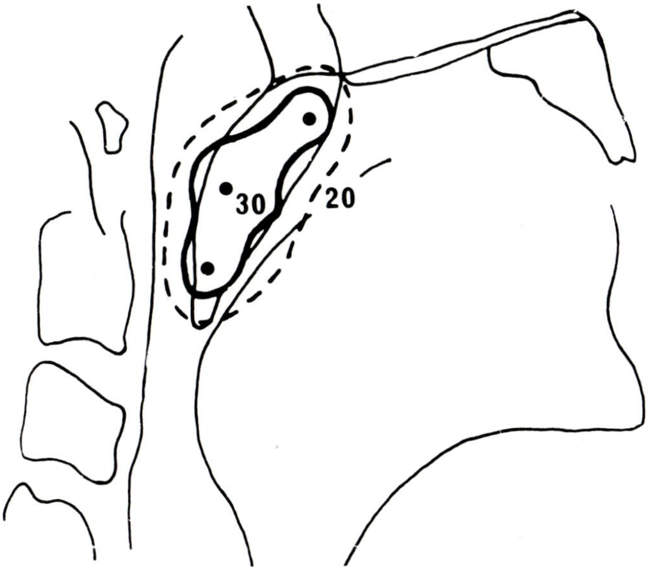

Figure 50.
c. Carcinoma of the soft plate. Graphic dosimetry taken from tomogram. Reference isodose x 30 rad/hr. for activity 1m Ci/cm.

Monitoring of the patient during the course of irradiation is quite simple, for this radioactive setup is usually well tolerated by the patient. The first 24 hours are rather uncomfortable because of the trauma caused by the anesthetic agent and the implantation which causes a painful temporary edema. The patient is maintained on analgesics and sedatives during this period.

Feeding remains possible, although the diet ought to be liquid in order to minimize the movements of the soft palate and to avoid its further traumatization by solid foods, which could also displace the radioactive material. The dietitian can be very helpful in this phase of the management of the patient. A lavage or a spraying of the oral cavity is carefully done two or three times a day.

Antibiotics can be given; their indication, however, remains optional for implantations of the soft palate, depending on the general condition of the patient, and especially on his pulmonary status.

The duration of irradiation naturally depends on the desired dose and the output of the radioactive setup. In a typical case, the dose rate is of the order of 50 to 60 rads/hour or 1200 to 1500 rads in 24 hours. The total duration of the irradiation is therefore, between three and six days for a total dose of 4000 to 7500 rads.

An alternate technique using curved guide gutters is possible, but seldom recommended. This technique requires vertical implantation and implies leaving the distal ends of the radioactive wires free in air, beyond the inferior border of the soft palate, which is very uncomfortable for the patient. This also results in an underdosage of the inferior half of the soft palate. Therefore, this alternate technique is only considered for lesions limited to the upper portion of the soft palate, perhaps extending slightly onto the hard palate.

c. *Therapeutic Results* [(1)] : Since 1959, we have treated 130 patients with this technique. In 51 cases followed for over three years, we have seen a rather mediocre survival rate of 27%. Most of these patients succumb to metastases, intercurrent disease or new primaries. We have observed only five local recurrences representing a 90% local control rate.

Tonsillar Region

a. *Clinical Anatomical Review:* The tonsillar region is a complex area containing several structures.

The boundaries of the tonsillar fossae are the anterior tonsillar pillars, the posterior tonsillar pillars and the glossotonsillar folds inferiorly. Although the fossae open widely inferiorly and posteriorly on the posterior surface of the oropharynx and the lateral wall of the pyriform sinuses, the lymphoid tissue of the true tonsil is located in their upper half.

Anteriorly, the mucous membrane covering the medial surface of the ascending ramus of the mandible represents a surface area varying considerably from one patient to another, and which is located between the anterior pillar and the retromolar trigone.

The close proximity of the tonsillar region to the soft palate above and to the base of the tongue below, establishes three areas clinically important in tumors of the tonsillar region:

1. Carcinomas of the tonsillar fossa proper and of the anterior and posterior pillars.
2. Carcinomas of the tonsillopalatine region that can extend to part of or to one half of the soft palate.
3. Carcinomas of the glossotonsillar region which can arise from the glossotonsillar fold and extend into the tonsillar fossa or into the base of the tongue.

In endotherapy, it is indispensible to be aware of the thickness of the soft tissues that separate the tonsillar region from the ascending branch of the mandible. In front of the anterior pillar and along the ascending branch of the mandible, the mucosa is in close proximity to the bone, while it is at a moderate distance from it at the level of the tonsillar fossa, or towards the posterior pillar. A transverse tomogram illustrates this anatomical finding by showing the oropharyngeal wall to be directed posteromedially with an angle of about 45° in relationship to the internal surface of the ascending branch of the mandible. The mucosa of the tonsillar region is directed obliquely upwards and medially forming a roof over the tongue. The result is that, with any implantation, the radioactive sources remain well separated from the bone in the upper and posterior region, while they come in close proximity to the bone and to the sensory nerves of the oral cavity (glossopharyngeal, lingual), inferiorly and anteriorly. The risk of radionecrosis and subsequent neuritis should, therefore, not be minimized when an implantation of the anterior portion of the tonsillar region is necessary.

b. Recommended Technique: We recommend the guide gutter technique of endotherapy (local anesthesia, sitting position).

Implantation of the Guides: Local anesthesia is achieved by injecting 5 to 10 cc of 1% Xylocaine at the mid portion of the anterior pillar infiltrating progressively the entire tonsillar region. Depending on the size of the lesion, 2 or 3 radioactive sources are used in a vertical or oblique direction implanting downward. If the point of entry is at the superior border of the tonsillar fossa, and if the inferior border of the soft palate joins the pharyngeal wall rather low, it may be necessary to insert the guide through the soft palate. In the case of a hairpin, the tonsillar fossa is easily framed by the anterior branch following the direction of the anterior pillar, or crossing it, while the posterior branch penetrates the thickness of the soft palate to follow the posterior pillar. A single hairpin, 3 or 4 cm long, is often sufficient to cover a small lesion of the tonsillar region, especially for residual tumor following teletherapy (Figure 51). For larger lesions, three radioactive sources are needed to cover the entire tonsillar region and to extend to the posterior oropharyngeal wall. In such cases it is advisable to place the hairpin posteriorly and a single pin anteriorly.

Insertion of the Radioactive Wires: By applying firm even traction on the plaque of the guides with nonserrated forceps, they are partially pulled out in order to bring their long axis in the direction of the mouth. The operator then introduces the radioactive pins, being careful to maintain this same orientation. With a reverse sliding motion, the radioactive material replaces the guides, which are removed, and nylon sutures are tied around the head of the pin.

The dosimetry, the monitoring of the application and the removal of the radioactive material follows the same rules described for the endotherapy of the soft palate.

Tonsillopalatine Region

In this region, the planes of the muscles and of the mucous membranes are oriented in different directions, and it is here that the hairpin guide technique has its most exclusive indications. This is because the parallelism of the two branches of the hairpin is maintained by the transverse branch of the pins despite the divergence of the tissue planes.

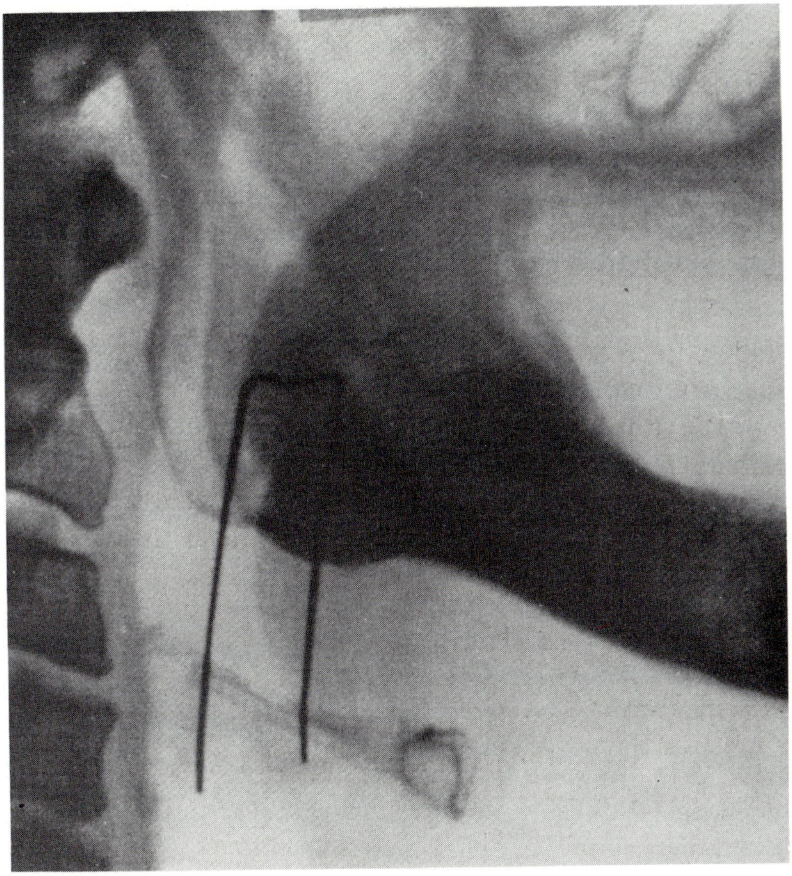

Figure 51. Carcinoma of the tonsil. A single hairpin 3 to 4 cm long is sufficient to irradiate a small lesion of the tonsillar fossa.

If the extent of the lesion on the soft palate is relatively small, a single plane of implantation is sufficient with the guides implanted downward and anteroposteriorly. The implantation is, therefore, started well up the mucosa of the soft palate, and the guides are pushed under the mucosa of the tonsillar fossa, or its posterior pillar, by guiding them with the finger and a mirror, in order to be assured that their points do not penetrate into the pharyngeal cavity.

If the soft palate is extensively involved, we recommend using two long curved single guides spaced at 12 mm, which are then after-loaded with a custom curved hairpin.

Glossotonsillar Region

The radioactive sources are placed on both sides of the glossotonsillar fold. Two parallel planes of irradiation are necessary, one in the pharyngeal wall and the other in the tongue. Thus, a box-shaped target volume is formed extending mostly toward the base of the tongue. The implantation of the pharyngeal guide does not present any significant difficulty. It is inserted first, downwardly and anteroposteriorly in the lower portion of the tonsillar region following the long axis of the glossotonsillar fold. The implantation of the glossal guide, is, on the contrary, more difficult and deserves detailed explanation. At rest and with the mouth closed, the dorsal surface of the tongue comes in contact with the hard and soft palate, curving laterally to come in contact with the pharyngeal wall and tonsillar region. During the implantation of the radioactive material, this topographic arrangement is altered by the forced opening of the mouth and the forward traction on the tongue. Thus, half of the base of the tongue to be treated is stretched and flattened anteriorly and medially. The mucosa that assumes a transverse orientation under the effect of traction, returns to a frontal or sagittal plane at rest, when the stretched muscle fibers resume their vertical curvature. The operator should, therefore, take into account this artificial alteration by traction, and assure a satisfactory position of the implantation when the tongue returns to rest. In practice, the glossal gutter guide is implanted in a sagittal direction on an axis oriented posteriorly and slightly laterally. Its medial branch then becomes the posterior or posteromedial source when the tongue returns to rest and the lateral source becomes anteriorly placed. As the guide is advanced, precautions are taken so that the points do not pierce the mucosa near the vallecula. In experienced hands, this implantation is rapidly accomplished. The radioactive pins are usually 4 cm long and occasionally 5 cm, especially when the lesion extends to the vallecula or to the aryepiglottic fold.

Therapeutic Results[2, 3] . All of our cases were squamous cell carcinomas. They were irradiated with telecobalt therapy or betatron therapy to a total dose of 4500 rads and subsequently received endotherapy with Iridium 192 to an additional 4000 rads at the reference isodose. In 143 patients followed for over 5 years, the following survival chart is obtained.

	NO	*N1*	*N2*	*N3*	*Total*	
T_1,T_2	16/27	7/22	0	5/26	28/75	37%
T_3	3/18	4/20	0	4/13	11/51	21%
T_3	1/7	3/8	0	0/2	4/17	23%
TOTAL	20/52	14/50	0	9/41	43/143	30%

Local recurrences have been uncommon in T_1 and T_2 lesions (6/75). They have been more numerous in the T_3 and T_4 categories (17/68). These results are not better than those achieved by external irradiation alone. This method of treatment is, therefore, reserved for special cases. Cases of serious necrosis have been observed only in treating extensively ulcerated lesions. Eight instances of necrosis have been noted, six of these occurred following treatment of a T_3 or T_4 lesion.

Base of Tongue

a. Clinical Anatomical Review: To precisely define the clinical anatomical borders of a cancer of the base of the tongue is difficult. The lateral limits of the base of the tongue are precise enough at the level of the glossotonsillar fold, however, the boundary of the base of the tongue is ill defined inferiorly at the vallecula, and especially anteriorly where it is in continuity with the mobile portion of the tongue without a distinct delineation. This clinical anatomical uncertainty is also reflected in the pathology of these tumors. In fact, many of the malignant tumors of the base of the tongue originate from adjacent structures. Subdivision of the different locations of these tumors is indispensible for clinical and therapy purposes. We will describe two regions, namely, centrally located lesions and those of the glossoepiglottic fold. The malignant tumors of the glossotonsillar region have already been described in this chapter (Figure 52).

Recommended Technique

1. Central Region of the Base of the Tongue — Superficial Lesions: We define superficial lesions as those which appear clinically to have no induration at depth, and which fail to show deep ulcerations on roentgenographic studies. They are essentially exophytic lesions. We recommend the guide gutter technique of endotherapy (local anesthesia, sitting position).

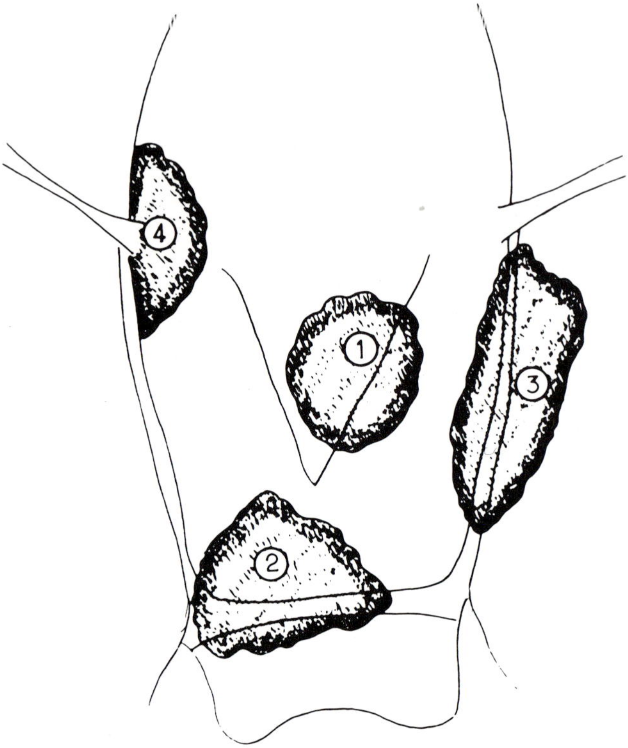

Figure 52. Carcinomas which involve the base of tongue. They may arise centrally (1) or from the vallecula (2) the glossotonsillar fold region (3) or from the junctional zone (4), (zone of the lingual junction of the anterior tonsillar pillar — palatoglossal fold).

Local anesthesia is achieved by using a lozenge of Tetracaine and a spray of 10% Xylocaine. When the gag reflexes disappear, 5 to 10 cc of 1% Zylocaine with adrenalin is infiltrated at one or two points just posterior to the circumvallate papillae infiltrating the anesthetic deeply into the muscles of the tongue. The implantation is accomplished through the oral cavity anteroposteriorly, and downwards corresponding to the sagittal axis of the tongue. The different radioactive sources are, therefore, distributed in a plane which is parallel to the mucosal surface of the base of the tongue. One hairpin is sufficient for small lesions. With three sources, nearly the entire base of the tongue can be covered, for example, with one hairpin and one single pin. The length of these is never less than 3 cm, and is more often 4 or 5 cm, especially if it is necessary to extend beyond the lower border of the vallecula (Figure 53). Points of entry of the guides depend on the anterior boundary of the lesion. A moderate degree of traction is maintained on the tongue at the time of implantation. The operator tries to maintain each guide a few mm beneath the mucosa, remaining parallel to the mucosal surface and without penetrating too deeply into the muscular layers of the tongue. It is also important not to come too close to the surface of the mucosa, especially at the vallecula. This position is checked with a mirror examination and radiographically.

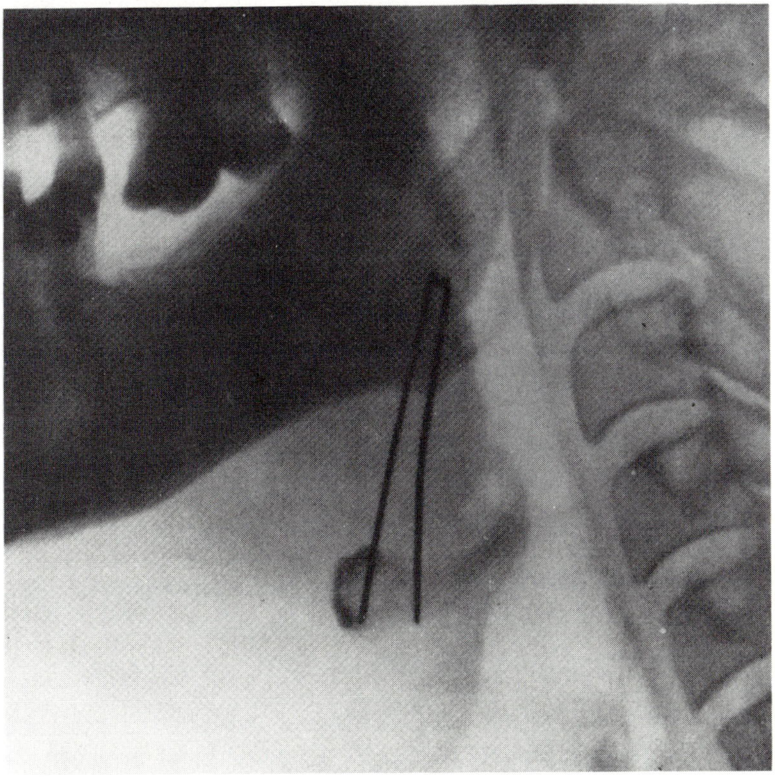

Figure 53. Cancer of Base of Tongue. A single long hairpin implanted in base of tongue and traversing the vallecular region for a superficial carcinoma of the central portion.

The radioactive material is usually well tolerated during the few days of the application. The patient can also take a liquid diet without great difficulty.

Infiltrating Lesions: The brachytherapist should delineate a rather large target volume encompassing the entire thickness of the base of the tongue and most of its length. We recommend the plastic tube technique of endotherapy (basal or general anesthesia, supine position, head extended). In principle, three or four radioactive loops open anteriorly are placed parallel to each other in a sagittal plane. Transversely, they will cover the entire base of the tongue or one affected side. Each branch of the loops penetrates the skin, the muscles and the mucosa, but its curved apex rests on the surface of the tongue (Figure 54).

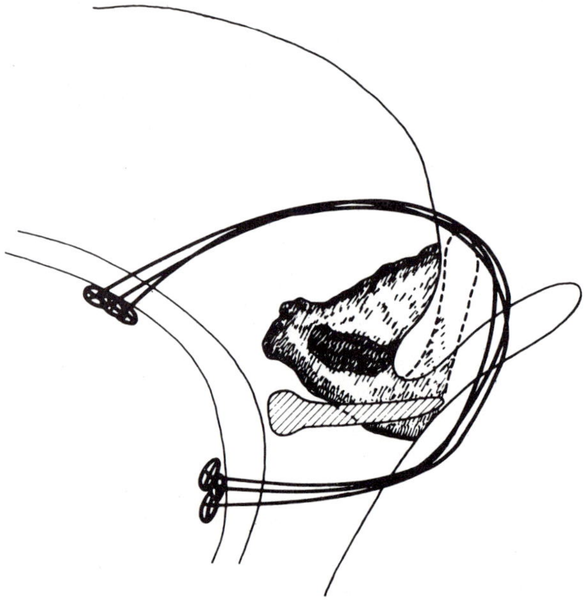

Figure 54. Cancer of glossoepiglottic region. Plastic tube technique. The loops encompass the epiglottis and pull it forward into contact with the base of tongue.

The brachytherapist and his assistants prepare the skin of the submental and cervical regions with antiseptic solutions. With one finger in the oral cavity, a drawing corresponding to the outline of the tumor is drawn on the skin with a dermatographic pencil. The surrounding areas are then draped with sterile towels.

Implantation of the Plastic Tubes

Each loop is placed according to the technique described in the chapter on technique (see page 33 and Figure 11 (a through e)). To form the loop, we systematically start with the inferior branch by implanting the guide needle either above or below the hyoid bone depending on the level of the lower border of the tumor as visualized on a lateral x-ray. The guide needle is introduced perpendicularly to the surface of the skin, while with the index finger of the free hand, the operator controls the penetration of the needle into the pharyngeal cavity. The spacing between each loop is controlled by the index finger, realizing that the width of the finger is about 15 to 20 mm and its thickness is about 12 to 15 mm. Immobilization buttons are then placed in their final position determined by the degree of traction applied on the tissues by each loop and after being assured that the target volume is covered as uniformly as possible. One can exert more traction on loops surrounding an area infiltrated by tumor, than on softer and less infiltrated tissues. After heparinizing each plastic tube, lead wires are introduced into each loop for dosimetry purposes.

When the patient recovers, usually the day following the implantation of the guide material, frontal and lateral roentgenograms are taken to locate the position of the target volume delimited by the inactive wires. With the use of these roentgenograms, one can establish the boundaries of the irradiation in relation to the surface of the skin, and also the respective lengths of the radioactive wires to be afterloaded into each loop. (Figure 55).

Loading of the Iridium 192 Wires: After the dosimetry has been calculated, afterloading is performed from behind lead screens. Depending on the ease with which the radioactive material slides into the tubes, one can use either a continuous wire or two wires introduced from either end, joining at the apex of the loop. With the use of fluoroscopy, their exact position is verified, and the radio active plastic tubes are fixed in the plastic guide tubes by crushing the immobilization buttons.

During the course of irradiation, the patient is maintained on antibiotics. Liquid feeding is accomplished either normally, which

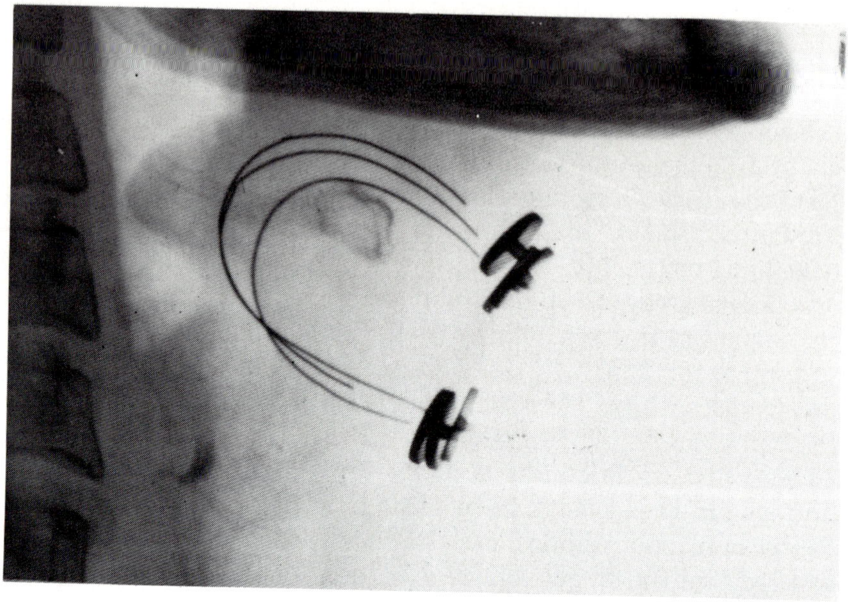

Figure 55. Cancer of Base of Tongue. Plastic tube technique. Dummy sources in portion.

is usually the case, or by nasogastric tube. With the use of analgesics and sedatives, this application is relatively well tolerated by all patients.

Special Consideration: If, because of a large tumor size, larger than usual loops are necessary, and are spaced by more than 20 mm, an underdosage in the middle of the target volume is unavoidable. In order to compensate for this, a transverse loop is added, the two branches of which are situated well within the target volume, equidistant from the other two rows. The apex of the loop is left inactive in order to avoid an overlap with the medial sagittal loop, which will otherwise create a hot area, that can produce radionecrosis of the base of the tongue.

2. Glossoepiglottic or Vallecular Region: In principle, irrespective of the size of the tumor, we recommend the plastic tube technique of endotherapy (basal or general anesthesia, supine position). This technique is essentially the same as the one used for the endotherapy of infiltrating lesions of the central portion of the base of the tongue.

The only difference is that the lower border of the target volume reaches the fixed portion of the epiglottis. The plastic tubes are introduced between the hyoid bone and the thyroid cartilages. The epiglottis is thus pulled towards and held against the base of the tongue and vallecula by the loops.

c. *Therapeutic Results:* From 1958 to 1967 we have treated 111 patients (4 T_1, 26 T_2, 51 T_3 and 30 T_4 lesions). The total five year survival is 17% (19/111). There have been 21 local recurrences. Most of these patients die of lymph node recurrences, metastases, intercurrent infection or from second primaries.

ORAL CAVITY

The indications for endotherapy with radium in this location have been long recognized, and its numerous successes cannot be contested. Artificial radioisotopes have, however, brought a substantial technical improvement for small lesions, where they can replace radium for greater comfort of the patient, and can be better used to treat advanced cases. In T_3 or T_4 lesions, teletherapy and/or chemotherapy is generally given prior to the endotherapy. For T_1 or T_2 lesions, initial teletherapy may also be given.

We will describe five different primary sites presenting different technical and biological problems, including the lips, the mucous membranes of the cheeks, the mobile portion of the tongue, the hard palate and the floor of the mouth.

Before describing the techniques of endotherapy for oral cavity lesions, it is indispensable to discuss the effect of irradiation on the teeth and the mandible. Devascularization of bone secondary to irradiation can precipitate necrotic complications following relatively low doses of about 4000 to 5000 rads. The mandible is particularly susceptible, especially when endotherapy is applied in its proximity. With these techniques, the irradiated area is usually small, but the dose of radiations is generally quite high in view of this proximity. With time, radionecrotic changes may become apparent at the level of the irradiated bone eventually extending to its medullary portion. This destructive process may result in a sequestrum that can be removed surgically, resulting in the complete healing of the remaining bone and overlying mucosa or it may progress and fracture the mandible, resulting in reinfection and fistula formation.

One ought not to exaggerate the development of bony complications. If the target volume of the endotherapy is sufficiently reduced, one is entitled to take certain risks of radionecrosis. These are in general limited to a small denudation of the bone or the elimination of small sequestra followed by a satisfactory healing of the tissues. It is also to be noted, that while in certain cases mandibular necrosis is not well tolerated by the patient, others are relatively well tolerated functionally, despite extensive involvement, and do not necessarily result in serious difficulties or malnutrition. The radiotherapist is capable of judging the calculated risks based on an accurate spatial dosimetry. The radioactive sources can sometimes be placed at a greater distance from the bony structures without jeopardizing an adequate dose at the level of the tumor.

In practice, two rules are followed every time endotherapy is considered in the oral cavity for lesions which are near the mandible:

1. Roentgenograms of the mandible are obtained to rule out possible pre-existing infiltration of the bone by tumor, in which case, endotherapy is quite risky, and abstention is advisable.

2. Once an indication for endotherapy is established, all poor teeth in contact with or at a short distance from the implant should be extracted. If several such teeth, and especially the molars, are to be extracted, general anesthesia followed by several days of rest is allowed for the recovery and complete healing of the gingival mucosa. Healthy teeth can either be extracted or preserved by special care (fluoride).

Lips

a. Clinical Anatomical Review: Both the upper and lower lips are divided into three zones; the skin of the lip, delimited by the inferior border of the nostril for the upper lip and by the labiomental groove for the lower lip. This zone is continuous with the vermilion surface delimited laterally by the oral commissures. The mucous membrane of the lips is delimited by the gingivolabial sulcus for both the upper and lower lips. In regard to tumor pathology, one zone deserves special mention, and that is the oral commissures, the point of origin of numerous squamous cell carcinomas. Anatomically, this commissural zone is defined arbitrarily as a circle 20 mm in diameter with its center at the commissure itself. Including, therefore, the lateral thirds of the upper and lower lips, as well as the adjacent zone of the cheek.

Apart from the commissural zone, carcinomas are most frequently found on the vermilion surfaces of the lower lip. One can also see numerous small carcinomas of the lip measuring only a few mm in diameter, one of the rare instances where T_1 lesions are seen frequently. Technically, we will consider three types of lesions: small lesions of the lower lip, large lesions of the lower lip and lesions of the commissure.

b. Recommended Technique

1. Small Lesions of the Lower Lip: We recommend the hypodermic needle technique of endotherapy (basal or local anesthesia, supine position). For lesions less than 1 cm in diameter a superficial transverse radioactive line on either side of the lesion is established. The length should be at least 2 cm if the target volume is to be sufficiently large. For larger lesions, this spacing is determined by the rules of the Paris system. The spacing of these lines is maintained by spacers cut to measure from small lengths of IV tubing. Dosimetry is usually by direct measurement. Because the lip is particularly tolerant of high doses of radiation, one can give more than 7000 rads at the isodose of reference, if necessary, to thoroughly irradiate portions of an exophytic tumor which may protrude above the plane of the implant.

The patient can be fed a liquid diet without difficulty. Mastication of solid foods should be forbidden since it could displace the needles.

The immediate reaction following this implantation, is a radioepithelitis with edema and ulceration of the mucosa. At the end of six weeks, a soft scar becomes apparent producing a discrete depigmentation of the mucous membrane with minimal retraction of the lip. Occasionally slightly nodular sclerotic changes are visible.

2. Large lesions of the Lower Lip: Three clinical characteristics are considered depending on whether the lesion extends concentrically, infiltrates in depth or extends on the surface transversely, as is frequently seen in lesions of the vermilion surface.

Concentrically Infiltrating Lesions: We recommend the hypodermic needle technique of endotherapy immobilized by plexiglass plaques (basal anesthesia, patient supine).

Implanting transversely, the hypodermic needles are introduced in the following order. The first needle is implanted submucosally slightly posterior to the junction of the vermilion surface and the labial mucosa. The second needle is implanted just anterior to the junction of the vermilion surface and the labial skin, and the third needle is located inferiorly and at a short distance above the labiomental sulcus. Thus, a triangular target volume is formed with its apex located inferiorly (Figure 56a).

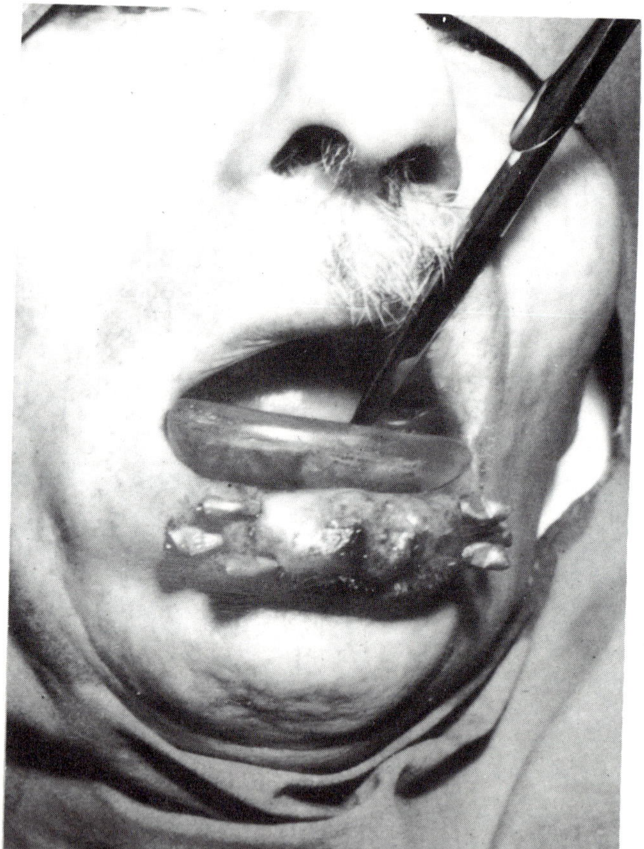

Figure 56. Cancer of the Lower Lip
a. Hypodermic needle technique. Plastic spacer between lip and gingiva.

The three needles are maintained strictly parallel to each other by two small plexiglass plaques perforated to accept them, and taped on the edges to avoid traumatizing the mucocutaneous junction. Depending on the choice of predrilled plaque, corrections of the implant are made automatically, establishing an optimal spacing between the three sources. The dosimetry is by direct measurement or from a sagittal tomogram made prior to afterloading the sources. The radioactive wires are introduced last (Figure 56b).

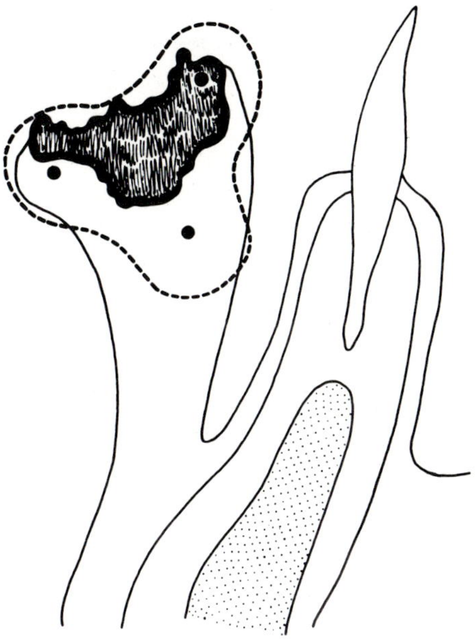

Figure 56. b. Diagram showing typical triangular target volume.

For lesions with transverse extensions on the surface, we recommend the plastic tube technique of endotherapy. These lesions are sometimes extensive and occupy about 2/3 of the vermilion surface (4 to 5 cm in length). This type of lesion often appears as a crusty ulceration, which is continuous with an area of nonulcerated hyperkeratosis showing no histological evidence of malignant change. Local anesthesia is possible should there by any contraindication to general anesthesia.

Two guide needles are implanted on a transverse axis, parallel to each other and covering the lesion anteriorly and posteriorly. The points of entry and exit are at least 5 mm beyond the apparent borders of the lesion. Plastic guide tubes are then substituted for the guide needles. Dosimetry is done in the usual manner and sources of the proper length are afterloaded.

Large and Infiltrating Lesions: We recommend a modification of the plastic tube technique in which large plastic tubes are not substituted for the guide needles which are themselves afterloaded with the inner tube. They are immobilized at their ends by plexiglass plaques or by pierced pieces of IV tubing.

These are uncommon lesions having extensive vegetating ulcerations extending onto the skin of the lip. The guide needles are always inserted along a transverse axis in 2 or 3 planes and immobilized. The guide needles are blocked at their exit from the skin by crushing immobilization buttons in place on the external surface of the corresponding plexiglass plaque, following which the points are cut off with pliers. (See Breast Technique for further details.)

3. Lesions of the Oral Comissure: Lesions of this type develop concentrically. They can extend to the upper as well as the lower lip, and occasionally to the adjacent cheek.

We recommend the plastic tube technique of endotherapy (basal anesthesia, supine position).

The implantation is done after disinfecting the skin. The projection of the target volume is drawn on the skin with a dermatographic pencil, superimposed on which a drawing of the desired radioactive lines is made. A single plane of implantation is usually sufficient. Generally 2 or 3 horizontal parallel radioactive sources are needed, their spacing depending on the vertical extension of the tumor. The spacing between each radioactive source is 12 to 15 mm and parallelism is established with the mouth closed. Starting superiorly and posteriorly, the needle penetrates the substance of the cheek, to emerge from the skin or mucous membrane of the upper lip. If three radioactive sources are used, the middle needle will protrude between the upper and lower lips, the exact exit point depending on whether the bulk of the tumor extends superiorly or inferiorly. The lower needle protrudes from the skin or mucous membranes of the lower lip. Outer plastic tubes are then substituted for the guide needles. Dosimetry is established on an oblique unidirectional tomogram taken perpendicularly to the radioactive sources. Finally, Iridium 192 wires are afterloaded and maintained in position with the metallic buttons.

In small lesions of the lower lip, no significant protection of the mandible is necessary in view of the small target volume. It is, however, advisable to extract nearby decayed incisor and canine teeth.

In treating larger lesions of the lower lip, it is advisable to first extract all decayed teeth and to use a plastic spacer that fits over the lower alveolar ridge in order to increase the distance between the lips and the mandible by about 15 to 25 mm. Thus, the dose to the anterosuperior region of the mandible can be diminished by about 15%. This apparatus also helps protect the tip of the tongue and the healthy lip minimizing uncomfortable reactions (Figure 56a).

For lesions of the commissure, systematic extractions of adjacent decayed teeth and use of a similar plastic spacer is advisable.

c. Thereapeutic Results: Since 1961, we have treated 115 epidermoid carcinomas of the lower lip with these techniques, of which 50 were new cases followed for more than three years. In this group, the local cure rate is 98% (3/3 for T_1, 22/22 for T_2,12/12 for T_3 and 12/13 for T_4). One ought to emphasize the excellent local results even in advanced lesions (Figure 57 (a,b). No serious complications were observed in these cases.

Lesions of the Buccal Mucosa

a. Clinical Anatomical Review: Carcinomas of the buccal mucosa are relatively uncommon. Endotherapy is easily adapted to the tumor volume for lesions of the buccal mucosa proper, while it is difficult, or even contraindicated, for lesions which are adjacent to the gingival mucosa or to the retromolar trigone. We will describe therapy techniques for three types of lesions: 1) small lesions of the buccal mucosa proper; 2) large lesions of the buccal mucosa proper; and 3) lesions of the gingivobuccal gutter.

b. Recommended Techniques

1) Very Small Lesions of the Buccal Mucosa: We recommend the guide gutter technique of endotherapy (basal anesthesia, supine position or local anesthesia, sitting position).

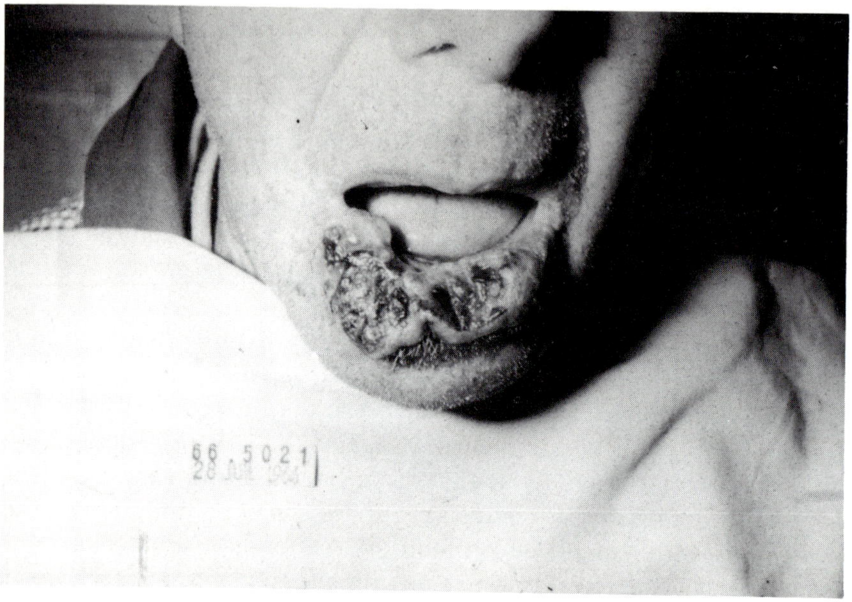

Figure 57. Squamous carcinoma lower lip, locally advanced.
a. Treated with 1^{192} hypodermic needle technique.
b. Same patient 3 years later.

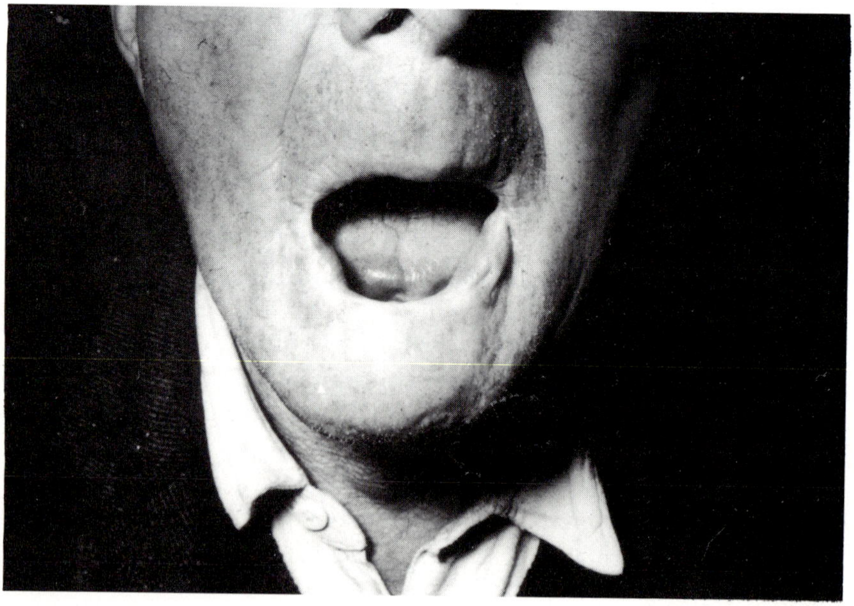

The boundaries of the tumor are established by palpation. The implantation of the guides is carried out in an anteroposterior direction using a double guide gutter without lip for two radioactive lines or a hairpin guide plus a single guide when three radioactive lines are needed. The tumor volume can generally be amply covered in a single plane. The length of the radioactive sources is about 3 cm. If a tomographic marker film is taken for dosimetry, the Vallebona movement yields the best results to eliminate the details on either side of the plane of implantation.

2) Moderately Large Lesions of the Buccal Mucosa Proper: We recommend the plastic tube technique of endotherapy (general anesthesia, supine position).

The endotracheal tube should be placed on the uninvolved side. The target volume is drawn on the skin with a dermatographic pencil while palpating the borders of the tumor. When the borders are in doubt, a fine needle piercing the cheek at several points can be used to mark the zone of the tumor on the corresponding skin of the cheek. The implantation of the guide needles is in a posteroanterior direction comparable to the technique used for lesions of the oral commissure (Figure 10). If the lesion is more than 2 cm thick, a second plane of implantation is necessary. The deeper plane covers the tumor at the level of the buccal mucosa, and the superficial plane, parallel to the former, is implanted just under the skin. The length depends on the extent of the tumor as projected on the skin of the cheek.

Frontal or oblique tomograms help establish the dosimetry.

3) Gingivobuccal Lesions: The majority of carcinomas of the buccal mucosa reach the gingivobuccal gutter or the retromolar trigone more posteriorly. When the lesions infiltrate the mandible or the maxillary region, endotherapy carries a high risk of radionecrosis of the underlying bone and cannot be recommended as a routine measure. It can, however, be used in combination with surgical excision, where endotherapy is only part of the treatment. The technique of implantation should be adapted to each case, and we do not prescribe a definite well-established technique for these cases.

c. *Therapeutic Results* (6) : Since 1960, we have treated 50 patients with these techniques. In a review made in 1966, we noted a three-year survival of over 50%; T_1 (7/12), T_2 (3/4), T_3 (2/4) and T_4 (2/4).

Mobile Portion of the Tongue

a. Clinical Anatomical Review: Squamous cell carcinomas are frequently noted to arise from the mobile portion of the tongue. The rather easy exteriorization of this structure, its rich vascularity and its remarkable tolerance to radiations make the indications of endotherapy quite predominant for lesions of this location. The techniques of implantation differ depending on whether the lesions are on the dorsal surface of the tongue, its borders or its ventral aspect. We will, therefore, consider successively infiltrating and noninfiltrating carcinomas of the dorsal surface of the tongue, where they rarely arise, of the lateral borders of the tongue, where they most often occur and of the ventral surface of the tongue. We will also consider large lesions which infiltrate a portion of the entire mobile tongue, often extending to the floor of the mouth or to the base of the tongue. As to the care of the teeth, they should be carefully attended to according to the principles described earlier.

b. Recommended Techniques

1) Dorsal Surface: Whether superficial lesions or larger infiltrating ulcerated lesions, the technique is the same, namely to encompass the lesion with parallel sources that penetrate the lingual muscles vertically.

We recommend the guide gutter technique of endotherapy (local anesthesia, sitting position).

Local Anesthesia: 1% Xylocaine with adrenalin is injected at three or four points around the lesion. These injections are made at depth within the muscles of the tongue, injecting 2 to 3 cc of anesthetic at each point. These multiple injections are necessary in view of the firm consistency of the lingual muscle inhibiting the easy diffusion of the anesthetic agent.

The Implantation of the Guides: The sitting position and the conscious state of the patient facilitate the application of the radioactive material. The tongue is pulled forward and out of the oral cavity without difficulty, and its inherent muscular tonicity is preserved, permitting an adequate control of the placement of the radioactive sources under normal physiologic conditions. Depending on the extent of the tumor, 4 to 6 radioactive sources surrounding the lesion are implanted using hairpin and single guides. Parallelism is verified by fluoroscopy and necessary corrections are made.

If the minimum diameter of the square or hexagon thus formed exceeds 3 cm, one or two radioactive sources are added in the center of the target volume to maintain homogeneity of dose. The clinical findings determine the length of the radioactive sources. For noninfiltrating lesions, 2 to 2.5 cm will be amply sufficient, while for an infiltrating lesion, it ought not to be less than 3 cm and may be 4 to 4.5 cm. Once the guides are in good position, nylon sutures are placed through the mucosa of the tongue beneath the heads of the guides. For hairpins, a deeper than usual suture is placed at the middle depression of the transverse branch.

Insertion of the Radioactive Wires: The most anterior guides are loaded first in order to be able to afterload the posterior-most guide in a field cleared of all other guides. Once the pins are substituted for the guide gutters, they are sutured to the mucosa (Figure 7 (a, b, c)).

After radiographic identification, the dosimetry is calculated from a transverse tomogram.

During such an application, the patient can take a liquid diet without difficulty. Only mild analgesics, frequent mouth washes and occasionally antibiotics are needed to maintain the patient in a functional and relatively comfortable state.

The ablation of this implant is somewhat more difficult than is usual in the oral cavity and oropharynx because of the deep suturing and the production of false membranes. Suction must be at hand. Great care must be taken to identify and firmly grip the sources prior to cutting the sutures and attempting to extract them.

About three weeks following the application, a marked radio-epithelitis appears, which is gradually replaced by a slightly depressed scar covered by a rather pale and smooth mucosa, which will persist indefinitely.

2) Noninfiltrating Lesions of the Borders of the Tongue: These lesions are usually vegetating at their periphery and centrally ulcerated. There is induration at their base for a thickness of only about 2 to 3 mm and their borders are well delineated. They usually arise from the middle third of the lateral margin of the tongue, and are usually ovoid in shape with the long axis in the sagittal direction. They vary in length between 1.5 and 3 cm. There are, however, exceptions to this general description.

We recommend the guide gutter technique of endotherapy (local anesthesia, sitting position).

The implantation of the guides is in the vertical direction, penetrating the dorsal surface of the tongue at its border and advancing them submucosally to the floor of the mouth. Two, three or four radioactive lines in "pallisade" cover part or all of the lateral margin of the tongue. The submucosal location of the guide is verified by palpation and fluoroscopic control. The tips of the guides can be seen at the floor of the mouth due to a slight lateral inclination during the implantation to avoid pushing them within the lingual muscle. The dosimetry is based on a transverse tomogram.

It is important to stress the fact that this technique of implantation in one plane should be reserved for superficial noninfiltrating lesions only. When the slightest infiltration is suspected clinically, even if only a few mm, it is advantageous to use another technique specifically developed for infiltrating lesions of the lateral border of the tongue.

3) Infiltrating Lesions of the Lateral Borders of the Tongue: In this section, we consider all lesions which infiltrate the lingual muscle, from the slightest infiltration to those infiltrating extensively, even to the midline of the tongue. Most of the squamous cell carcinomas of the tongue are in this group.

We recommend the guide gutter technique of endotherapy (local anesthesia, sitting position).

Two considerations are made depending on the extent of the infiltration.

(1) If the infiltration is less than 1.2 cm, the implantation is achieved by the "en cavalier" horseback technique of placing two or three hairpin guides in a row from front to back. Oriented transversely, they are implanted vertically, starting at the dorsum of the tongue. There results a target volume encompassed by a superficial row of radioactive sources formed by the lateral branches of the pins, and of a deep row from the medial branches of the pins. (Figure 10)

If three hairpin guides are needed, the anterior most is inserted first, and is the most critical considering its proximity to the ventral surface of the tongue, and to the medial surface of the mandible. The posterior most one is inserted next, and the middle one is placed last under televised fluoroscopic control, and its parallelism corrected until it is equidistant from the two distal guides. By palpating the position of the lips of the guides, their relation to the mucosa of the floor of the mouth is checked. For larger lesions, an extra single guide is occasionally added at the anterior border of the target volume, usually near the tip of the tongue along its ventral surface.

(2) If the infiltration exceeds 1.2 cm, the implantation is initially carried out according to the same rules as above. In addition, a sagittally oriented hairpin guide is added slightly to the opposite side of the midline of the tongue, at the point where the tumor infiltrates most deeply.

When the radioactive setup is correct, the sutures are placed, and Iridium 192 pins are substituted for the guides. The length of these sources depends on the size of the tumor, usually varying between 4 to 5 cm, total length.

4) Ventral Surface: Only those lesions confined to the ventral surface of the tongue without extension to the floor of the mouth are considered here. Lesions affecting both locations will be discussed in the chapter on Floor of the Mouth.

We recommend the guide gutter technique of endotherapy (local anesthesia, sitting position).

The implantation is achieved in a plane parallel to the mucosa and under conditions similar to those for noninfiltrating lesions of the lateral margins of the tongue. Two or four radioactive lines are sufficient to cover part or the entire ventral surface of the tongue.

The dosimetry is based on a transverse or frontal oblique tomogram.

5) Massively Infiltrating Lesions: These lesions reach or extend beyond the midline of the tongue and infiltrate its deep muscles to a greater extent than those lesions already discussed. They can also infiltrate the floor of the mouth and extend into the base of the tongue. This type of lesion and results of treatment by the plastic tube technique of endotherapy, are discussed in the following chapter on the Floor of the Mouth.

Floor of the Mouth

a. Clinical Anatomical Review: Strictly speaking, the floor of the mouth consists of all the soft parts encompassed within the mandibular arch, including the tongue. However, in clinical cancer terminology, the floor of the mouth is limited to a horseshoe shaped, horizontal gutter, delimited medially and posteriorly by the tongue and laterally and anteriorly by the mandible. This structure varies in width from 5 to 15 mm and is covered by a very thin mucous membrane. Squamous cell carcinomas of the floor of the mouth are rather frequently seen. Because of the narrow space, these tumors readily extend towards the lower gingival mucosa laterally and towards the tongue medially.

We will successively discuss the endotherapy of lesions limited to the floor of the mouth, lesions at its junction with gingival mucosa and lesions of the junction of the floor of the mouth with the tongue.

b. Recommended Techniques

1) Lesions of the Floor of the Mouth: These are usually lesions which are only slightly infiltrating, extending more or less lengthwise, and usually located in the anterior half of one side of the floor of the mouth. They do not extend to the gingival mucosa or to the tongue.

We recommend the guide gutter technique of endotherapy (local anesthesia, sitting position).

After applying a contact anesthetic on the entire mucosal surface of the oral cavity, and after injecting local anesthesia at the site of the implantation, the double guide gutters are inserted vertically on both sides of the lesion in a plane perpendicular to the long axis of the floor of the mouth or to the medial surface of the mandible. The obliquity of the implantaion increases as the width of the floor of the mouth decreases. It is, however, important to keep a double plane of implants encompassing the medial and lateral borders of the lesion. Occasionally, it will be necessary to complete this implantation with a single guide in front of or behind the edges of the lesion. For example: two hairpins and a single guide for a lesion measuring 2 to 2.5 cm in length and 6 to 8 mm in width. The guides are 3 cm long and their parallelism is checked with the image amplifier. Wide nylon sutures are gently placed under their heads. Lastly, the radioactive sources are substituted for the guides starting with the anteriormost one. The length of the radioactive sources depends on the thickness of the lesion, but should never be less than 2 cm long. Dosimetry is calculated from a transverse tomogram, establishing with great precision the exact position of the wires at different levels and their relationship to the medial surface of the mandible. It is important to know the position of the reference isodose with respect to the mandibular bone because of the risk of radionecrosis.

During the application, the ventral or lateral surfaces of the tongue rest on the heads of the radioactive sources with no separating materials interposed. The patient is usually quite comfortable during the application requiring little analgesia, and he is able to take a liquid or semisolid diet.

When the application is completed and after the radioepithelitis has subsided, the mucosa of the floor of the mouth is practically normal, although one often sees some degree of fibrosis of substitution proportional to the size of the original tumor. When radionecrotic changes of the floor of the mouth are suspected within a few months following the irradiation, these changes should be differentiated from a recurrence of tumor by biopsy.

2) Lesions of the Junction of the Floor of the Mouth and the Gingival Mucosa: These are usually lesions of the floor of the mouth extending to the gingival mucosa. If the mandibular bone is clinically or radiographically involved by tumor, it is advisable to avoid using radiotherapy, since necrotic changes following such treatment is very common. In these cases, an extensive surgical excision en bloc is more advisable. If the lesion of the gingival mucosa does not involve the bone, or when surgery is contraindicated, endotherapy alone can be used with caution. It may also be considered if the lesion is small and does not necessitate using more than two radioactive lines lying near the mandible.

3) Lesions of the Junction of the Floor of the Mouth with the Tongue: In general, the more infiltrating squamous cell carcinomas of the floor of the mouth usually extend towards the tongue. Sometimes these lesions are relatively small, developing similarly to an opened book with the ulceration and growth extending symmetrically on the floor of the mouth and the ventral surface of the tongue. In other cases, the origin of the tumor is impossible to determine when the tumor has infiltrated widely.

Small Lesions: We recommend the guide gutter technique of endotherapy (local anesthesia, sitting position).

The technique of implantation in these cases is similar to the technique used for infiltrating lesions of the borders of the tongue. It is, therefore, an implantation "en cavalier," with slight obliquity.

The medial branches are situated well within the lingual muscles beyond the medial edge of the tumor, and the lateral branches are implanted into the floor of the mouth at the lateral border of the tumor. For lesions involving the anterior portions of the floor of the mouth, and considering the dose in relation to the medial surface of the mandible, the lateral or the anterior radioactive sources are placed within a few millimeters of the gingvia, implanting them within tumor, if necessary. On the lingual side, one should not hesitate to place the medial branches well beyond the boundaries of the tumor. The reason for this consideration is that the extension of the tumor laterally and anteriorly is usually limited by the natural barrier provided by mandible, while it extends without difficulty into the muscles of the tongue, where tumor is often found beyond the clinically palpable lesion. Pins 3 to 4 cm in length are used, and the retaining sutures should always be placed well within the muscles of the tongue.

Massively Infiltrating Lesions: We recommend the plastic tube technique of endotherapy (general anesthesia, supine position).

Irrespective of the clinical extension of the tumor and the usual predominance of the lesion on one side or the other, the principle of the implantation should take into account the trapezoidal shape of the mandibular arch. Five vertical radioactive sources in two planes with a posterior row of three sources and an anterior row of two sources are usual (Figure 58). This basic setup could be slightly inclined in a right or left oblique plane, depending on the lateral extension of the lesion, and if necessary a sixth source can be added.

The patient receives nasotracheal anesthesia. The oral cavity is kept open with a rubber retractor placed on the side least involved by the tumor. A projection of the tumor and the points of entry of each guide needle are drawn on the skin of the submental and submaxillary regions. The skin and oral cavity are then prepared with antiseptic solution.

Three looped plastic tubes are placed in sagittal or parasagittal planes. The medial loop is inserted first in order to immobilize the tip of the tongue in a mid-line position. The anterior guide needle is inserted first. Starting at the skin and shaving the internal surface of the mandibular symphysis, it makes its exit on the dorsal surface of the tip of the tonue. The posterior needle is placed at the posterior

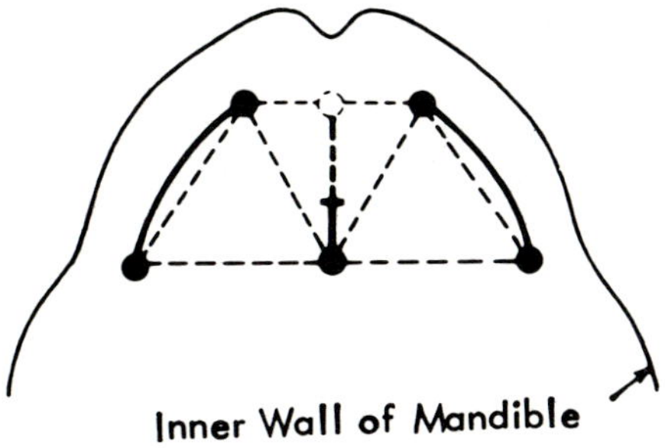

a

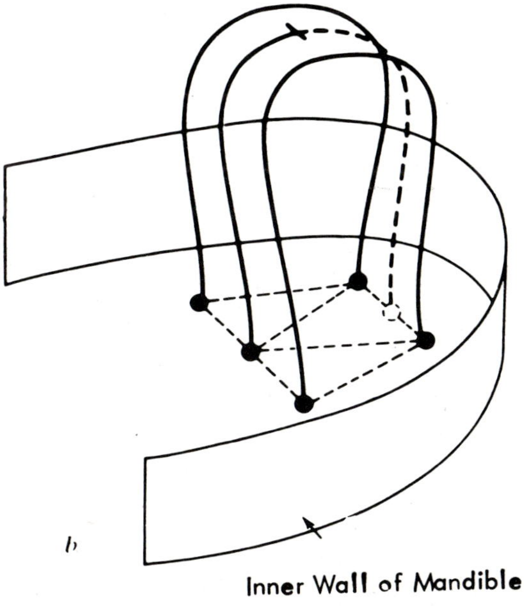

b

Figure 58. Carcinoma of Floor of Mouth. Plastic tube technique for locally advanced lesion. Selective loading of only the posterior branch of the central loop.

border of the tumor near the center of the mobile portion of the tongue. Then the outer tube is inserted by introducing the first branch of the loop with the posterior needle according to the technique previously described (Raynal's technique). The right and left lateral loops are then placed with the same technique, allowing a few mm distance between the plastic tubes and the mandibular bone. The two lateral loops diverge slightly posteriorly and laterally, but remain parallel to the horizontal branches of the mandible.

The three posterior branches are separated from each other by a distance of 1.5 to 2 cm, while the distance between the loops remains less than 2 cm. At the end of this procedure, three posterior and two anterior radioactive sources are introduced by using all three branches of the posterior loops and only the two lateral branches of the anterior loops. The middle anterior tube is not afterloaded and serves only the purpose of fixation (Figure 58).

If the spacing between the two anterior and posterior planes exceeds 2.5 cm, a transverse loop is added. Its relation to the other radioactive sources is according to the same principles of implantation as for large tumors of the base of the tongue.

If the extension of the tumor is definitely greater on one side, the homologous lateral loop is off set posteriorly, and all six branches of the three loops are used (Figure 59 (a, b, c)).

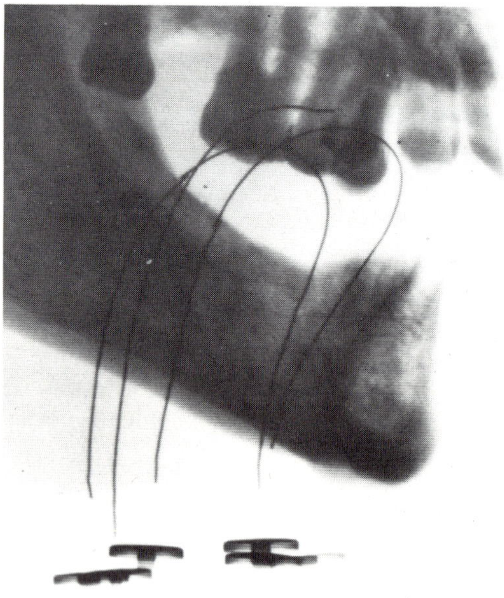

Figure 59. Carcinoma of the Floor of Mouth.
a. Dummy sources in position. Lateral view.

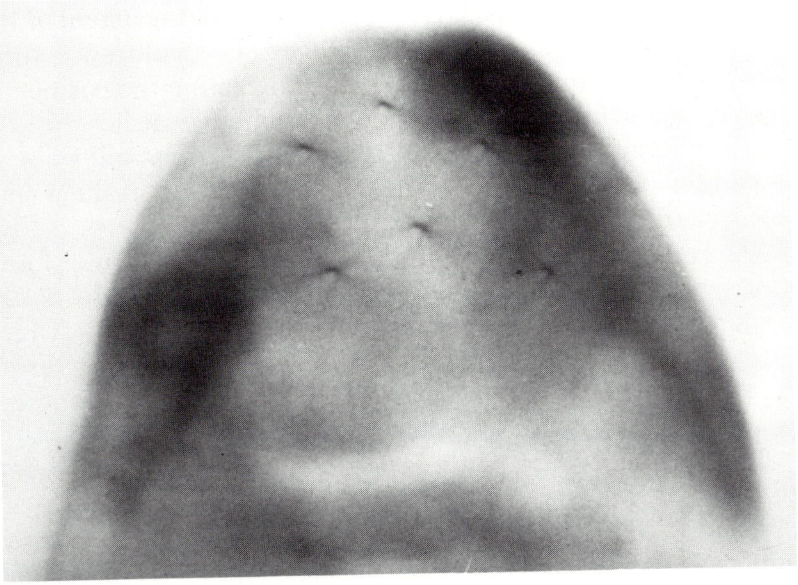

Figure 59. b. Carcinoma of the Floor of Mouth. Tomogram.

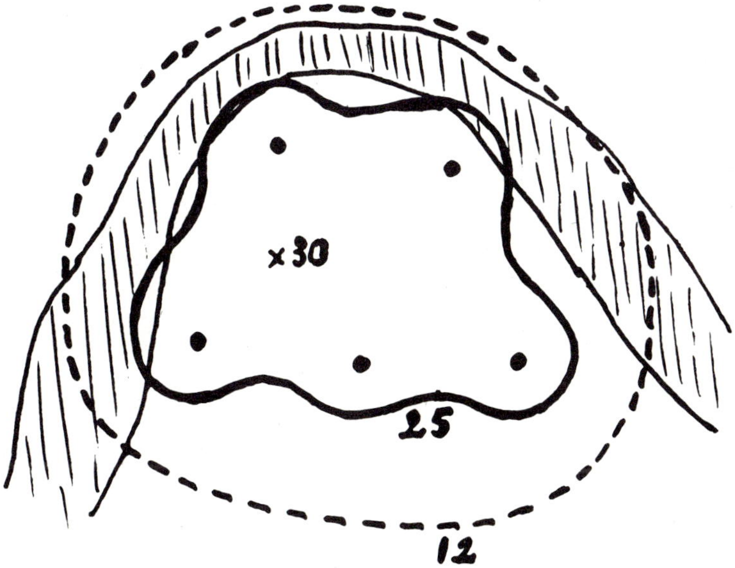

Figure 59. c. Carcinoma of the Floor of Mouth. Representative dosimetry taken from tomogram.

The length of each radioactive loop varies with the extent of the tumor towards the skin. The dosimetry is calculated from a transverse tomogram by computer, carefully noting the position of the reference isodose in relation to the mandibular arch.

This implantation is usually well tolerated by the patient who can take a liquid diet, and even if there is much discomfort, feeding via a nasogastric tube is still possible.

In the months following the application, close clinical and radiographic followup of the patient and the mandible are important to rule out the development of osteoradionecrosis, which is always possible despite all precautions. These complications are of special consideration in view of the large target volume encompassed by the mandibular arch.

c. *Therapeutic Results:* Since 1959, we have treated 407 patients with these techniques. All of these cases were squamous cell carcinomas, and most were well differentiated. We have included all carcinomas of the soft tissues included within the mandibular arch, including, therefore, lesions of the mobile portion of the tongue and floor of the mouth. The treatment techniques and the prognosis of lesions affecting these two areas are identical. We have classified these lesions into 5 groups depending on size:

T_1 : Noninfiltrating tumors less than 1 cm in diameter

T_2A : Noninfiltrating tumors 1 to 2 cm in diameter

T_2B : Tumors 2 to 3 cm in diameter infiltrating to a depth of up to 1 cm.

T_3A : Tumors 3 to 4 cm in diameter infiltrating to a depth of up to 1.5 cm.

T_3B : Tumors 4 to 5 cm in diameter infiltrating for a depth of up to 2 cm.

T_4 : Tumors exceeding 5 cm in diameter and infiltrating at a depth of up to 2 cm.

239 of the total of 407 patients were new cases followed for more than 2 years. The 2-year local control is as follows:

T_1	: 13/13	T_3A	: 50/54
T_2A	: 37/38	T_3B	: 49/63
T_2B	: 45/48	T_4	: 15/23

Local recurrences are rare in lesions 3 cm or less in diameter. The survival rate is, however, severly affected by the presence or the subsequent development of lymphadenopathy or intercurrent diseases. The overall 3-year survival rate is about 40%. Severe necroses developed in 10% of the patients, being more frequent as the size of the lesion increased. Numerous other minor acceptable necroses were seen which healed with appropriate treatment.

The Hard Palate

a. Clinical Anatomical Review: Carcinomas of the hard palate are rarely seen. Those which occur are usually squamous cell carcinomas, although occasional adenocarcinomas or cylindromas are encountered. The indications of endotherapy are reserved for lesions which involve only the mucosa of the palate and do not extend to the underlying bone. These indications are, therefore limited to the small T_1 or T_2 lesions, but for these endotherapy is well indicated.

b. Recommended Technique: We recommend the guide gutter technique of endotherapy (local anesthesia, sitting position).

The concave shape of the palate necessitates the use of curved guides. The axis of implantation is in a sagittal or parasagittal direction.

Local anesthesia is administered at two or three points, pushing the anesthetic rather forcefully in order to detach the mucosa from the underlying bone. This detachment is produced all along the predicted length of the radioactive sources.

In this location, single guide gutters are used to good advantage. The first guide is introduced into the submucosa using forceps to hold the head of the guide rather tightly. A second guide is introduced parallel to the first and spaced at a distance of 8 to 15 mm. Their parallelism is controlled with the image amplifier. Despite the detachment of the mucosa, the guides can be stopped by the underlying bone because of possible deformities of the bone or any accentuation of its concavity. By moving them slightly from side to side, these difficulties can be overcome. Two radioactive lines are usually sufficient to encompass these rather small lesions.

The Iridium 192 wires are then introduced and substituted for each guide, after having curved them slightly to match the concavity of the palate. The looped head of each wire is oriented laterally so that no overdosage results on either side of the anterior border of the target volume. A nylon suture is passed under the mucosa in an anteroposterior direction slightly behind the head of each radioactive wire.

The dosimetry is based on a frontal tomogram.

The application is functionally well tolerated.

In the months following the application, necrosis of the mucosa which surrounded the head of each radioactive source can appear, sometimes denuding the underlying bone over small areas a few mm in diameter. These areas remain limited, however, and produce no significant functional difficulty. When the target volumes are small, osteoradionecrosis of the palate is uncommon.

c. Therapeutic Results: Since 1961, we have treated 9 cases (3 T_1 and 6 T). We have observed only one local recurrance. Four cases have had local necrosis limited to the mucosa surrounding the heads of the radioactive sources which subsequently healed with no functional consequences.

REFERENCES

1. Pierquin, B., Chassagne, D., Issa, P., et Vandenbrouck, C.: L'éndocuriethérapie des carcinomas épridérmoides du voile par l' Iridium 192, J. de Radiologie, *50:*23-27, 1969
2. Pierquin, B., Raynal, M., Ennuyer, A., et Bataini, P.: Etude comparative des résultats concérnant les épithéliomas de la region amygdalienne traités a l'Institût Gustave Roussy et á la Fondation Curie, *Annales de Radiologie, 9:*815-824, 1966.
3. Raynal, M., Piérquin, B., Chassagne, D., et Raventos, E.: Résultats concérnant 133 cas d'épitheliomas de la region amygdalienne surdoses par endocuriethérapie avec Iridium 192, *J. de Radiologie, 51:*532, 1970.
4. Mouzon (A): "La curiethérapie avec préparation non radio-active dans les cancers de la base de langue." These pour le Doctorat en Médecine. Paris-Creteil — 1973.
5. Pierquin, B — Chassagne, D — Pieter, E — Raynal, M — Baillet, F — "L'endocuriethérapie par Iridium 192 des carcinomas épidérmoides de la lèvre inférieure." *Journal de Radiologie — 53:*207-212, 1972.
6. Pierquin, B., Chassagne, D., et Quint, R.: L'endocuriethérapie des carcinomas épidérmoides de la face interne de la joue, *Annales d'Oto-Laryngologie, 84:*403-408, 1967.
7. Pierquin, B., Chassagne, D., Cachin, Y., Baillet, F., et Fournelle Le Bruis, F.: Carcinomas épidérmoides de la langue mobile et du plancher buccal, *Acta Radiologica, 9:*465-480, 1970.

8. Pierquin, B., Chassagne, D., Baillet, F., and Castro, J. R.: The place of implantation in tongue and floor of mouth cancer, *J. A. M. A.*, *215:*961-963, 1971.

HYPOPHARYNX

The hypopharynx is an anatomical region where numerous malignant tumors arise, consisting of the laryngeal structures, the piriform sinuses, the epiglottis and the various folds which join these structures. Despite many different reports, brachytherapy has never played a major role in the treatment of squamous cell carcinomas of this region. There are three main reasons for this relative lack of therapeutic indications. Firstly, the physical conditions for external irradiation are excellent at the level of the neck since hypopharyngeal lesions are always at a short distance from the skin and are easily localized externally. Moreover, limited or radical surgery, including a total laryngectomy, can produce very satisfactory results. Finally, the risk of chondronecrosis or intractable edema of the laryngeal structures is high when radioactive sources are placed inside it, or in contact with the cricoid, thyroid or arytenoid cartilages.

In view of these considerations, indications for brachytherapy in the hypopharynx are limited to lesions located above the larynx, namely, the epiglottis or the arypharyngoepiglottic region.

Epiglottis and Arypharyngoepiglottic Region

a) Clinical Anatomical Review: These are squamous cell carcinomas of the free border of the epiglottis or the arypharyngoepiglottic region extending to the pharyngoepiglottic, aryepiglottic or the lateral glossoepiglottic folds. Brachytherapy can be achieved under good technical conditions for lesions which extend predominantly towards the epiglottis or the valleculae, while it is restricted for lesions which extend predominatly towards the pharyngeal walls.

b) Recommended Technique: We recommend the plastic tube technique of endotherapy (basal anesthesia, supine position).

The basic principles of this technique have already been described for malignant tumors of the base of the tongue and the vallecular regions. We should, however, emphasize that the loops should be as small as practical to avoid including a large area of the base of the tongue. If the lesion extends to the pharyngeal wall, the most lateral loop is placed within the wall itself, bringing the plastic tube onto the surface of the mucosa only at the apex of the loop.

It is also important to remember that when the free portion of the epiglottis is involved by tumor, immobilization of the epiglottic cartilage by the corresponding loops is necessary in order to keep the free portion of the epiglottis within the target volume.

c) Therapeutic Results: We have treated only a very small number of patients with carcinomas of the epiglottis or the arypharyngoepiglottic region with this technique. It is our experience, however, that the brachytherapeutic indications deserve to be developed further, especially for small superficially infiltrating lesions.

Special Consideration

Particular endotherapeutic indications are to be considered for recurrent lesions around tracheostomy openings following total laryngectomies. We have treated four such cases, either with plastic tubes or guide gutters, achieving local control in three.

REFERENCE

1. Ledman, M; Place of Radiotherapy in treatment of cancer of larynx, *Brit. Med. J., 1:*1639-1646, 1961.

Cervical Adenopathies

a. Clinical Anatomical Review: The indications for endotherapy of cervical adenopathies are essentially related to the contraindications of the other therapeutic modalities, whether surgery or radiation therapy. Clinically, these are usually metastatic lymphnodes from squamous cell carcinomas arising in the upper aerodigestive passages. Occasionally, no primary lesion is found, and in some cases, they may be metastatic manifestations of epithelial malignancies originating in other primary sites.

They may also represent residual cancer that the surgeon could not extirpate at the level of the carotid arteries, and in other cases surgery may have been contraindicated because of advanced age, poor general condition or other factors. More often, they are recurrent disease in lymph nodes following previous surgery and/or teletherapy.

In any event, endotherapy may be widely indicated irrespective of the volume of tumor to be irradiated, with two exceptions, namely, lesions associated with extensive edema and inflammatory change, and those with deeply ulcerated areas which may involve a high risk of hemorrhage from the carotid arteries. It is important to note, that postoperative endotherapy is performed only after any surgical scar has healed completely, usually 10 to 15 days following the operative procedure.

b. Recommended Technique: We recommend the plastic tube technique of endotherapy (basal or general anesthesia, supine position).

Two methods can be considered:

1. Technique with Straight or Curved Sources. This technique is recommended for all superficial or deep adenopathies which do not extend to the underlying mucosa. The axis of implantation is oriented inferiorly and anteriorly, parallel to the cutaneous folds. Depending on the thickness of the target volume, this implant contains one, two or three planes; if the thickness exceeds 2 cm, at least two planes are necessary. For the deeper planes and for retromandibular adenopathies, it is more convenient to use a long curved surgical hook instead of straight guide needles, to allow the plastic tubes to slide around the deeper surfaces of the adenopathy. When the surgical hook appears through the skin, the outer plastic tube is pushed firmly onto its point. The extraction of the surgical hook carries the plastic tube into position (Figure 60 (a, b, c)).

Technique of Loops Embracing the Mucous Membranes

This technique is recommended for deep lying adenopathies which displace the pharyngeal mucosa in the retromandibular region. These are generally very large lesions.

At the level of the retromandibular region, the loops are placed horizontally with their posterior branches along the cervical spinal column, and their anterior branches along the medial surface of the ramus of the mandible. This positioning will, therefore, encompass the vascular and lymphatic plexus of the superior carotid region.

The dosimetry is based on tomograms. Despite previous full course teletherapy, an additional 7000 rads can be added to the

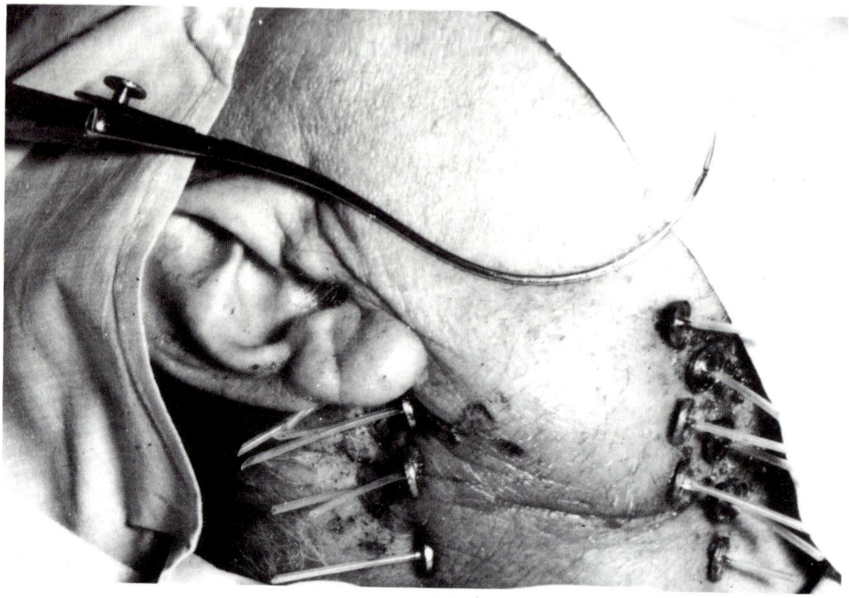

Figure 60. Brachytherapy of cervical lymphadenopathies.
a. Retromandibular area. Surgical hook used to deeply implant plastic tubes.

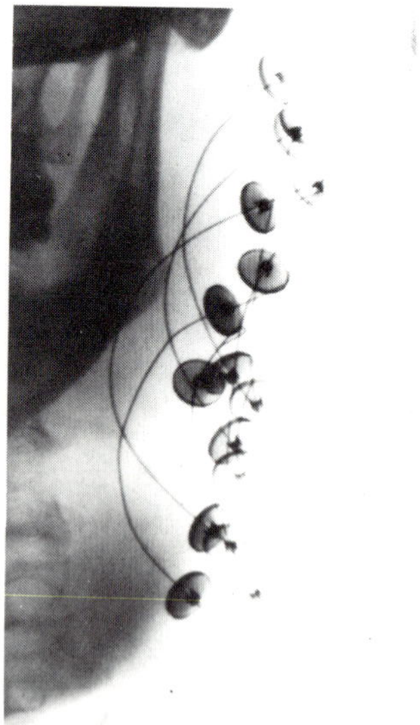

Figure 60.
b. Same case. Frontal roentgenogram.

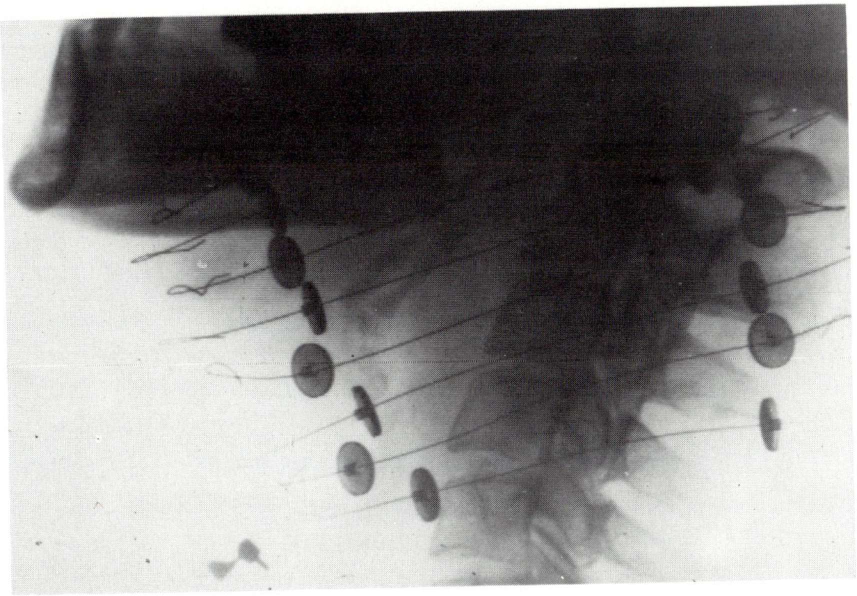

Figure 60.
c. Same case. Lateral roentgenogram.

reference isodose without risk of necrosis, provided that the skin is in good condition without deep ulcerations initially.

At the time of the removal of the radioactive setup, one should anticipate the possibility of a carotid artery hemorrhage. It is not unusual to find that one or two plastic tubes have pierced the external or internal carotid arteries without producing functional inconveniences. The plastic tubes are removed slowly, branch by branch, starting from above and alternating sides. Effective suction should be at hand. If any bleeding sites are seen, this can always be stopped by applying firm constant manual pressure for a few minutes.

a. Therapeutic Results: Since 1960, we have treated 210 patients with this technique. 124 cases have been observed for over three years in which group we noticed a complete disappearance of adenopathy in 31 cases and a significant regression in 40 cases. The other patients had poor results or were lost to follow-up. The best results are with metastatic adenopathies related to squamous carcinomas of the oropharynx. In essence, this treatment is palliative, taking into account previous therapeutic attempts and additional risks. It is, however, of great interest that significant palliation was accomplished in the majority of instances.

REFERENCES

1. Pierquin, B., Raventos, A., et Chassagne D.: L'endocuriethérapie des adenopaties cervicales malignes par Iridium 192, *J. de Radiologie, 51:*237-240, 1970.

Chapter VIII

THE SKIN

The indications for endotherapy and plesiotherapy are numerous and varied for lesions of the skin. Techniques have recently been developed using artifically radioactive elements which have widened the scope of plesioelectron therapy and endophoton therapy[1]. For all lesions less than 1 mm thick, plesioelectron therapy with either P^{32} or Sr^{90} is recommended. For thicker lesions, we recommend endotherapy with Iridium 192.

KELOIDS

a. Clinical Anatomical Review: Keloids present as a firm tumefaction within the dermis in areas which have been traumatized by surgery, burns, abscesses, etc. These lesions are fibromas several mm thick which protrude above the surface of the skin. This fibromatous tissue has proven to be quite radiosensitive in the first few days or weeks of its formation. Teletherapy and endotherapy share indications for the treatment of this condition.

b. Recommended Technique[2]*:* We recommend the hypodermic needle or plastic tube technique of endotherapy using Iridium 192 wires (local or general anesthesia).

The implantation is made during the same operative procedure, following surgical excision of the keloid.

A hypodermic needle is sutured into position between the edges of the wound with ultrafine synthetic sutures. These sutures are placed strictly within the dermis (Figure 61).

In practice, sutures are placed at intervals of 5 mm, with every fifth suture placed more deeply to hold the needle. The epidermis is left intact and is not pierced by any of these sutures. It is then approximated with micropore adhesive tape only.

The two ends of the hypodermic needle protrude beyond the ends of the wound by 5 mm and are separated from the underlying skin by small segments of leaded rubber to protect it from any unnecessary irradiation.

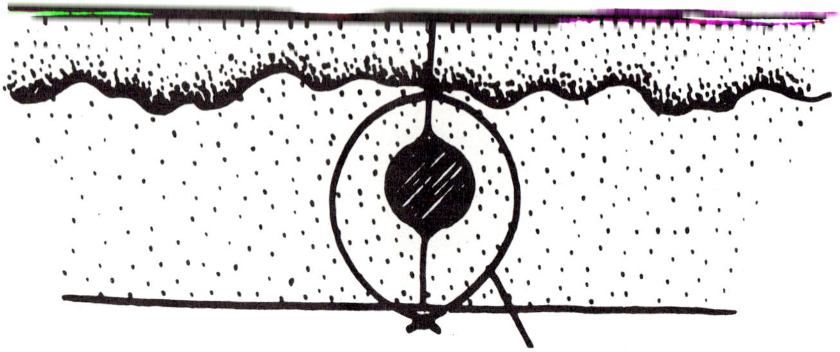

Figure 61. Keloids. Sutures are not allowed to pierce the epidermis.

Rigorous precautions are adhered to, in order to prevent any subsequent inflammation. The usual aseptic conditions are necessary. Catgut sutures and electrocoagulation are avoided and hemostasis is obtained by simple compression with gauze soaked in adrenalin and by the dressing itself. Irritant suture material such as silk and wool are also to be avoided.

To avoid the formation of a hematoma, which acts as a foreign body between the lips of the wound, a piece of gauze soaked in normal saline is kept on top of the micropore closure and held in place by adhesive tape.

The ends of the needles are allowed to protrude from the dressing. The radioactive material is usually inserted 3 to 4 hours after the surgical intervention. After removing the inactive stylet from the needle, the Iridium 192 wire is inserted directly into the needle. This wire has a diameter of 0.3 mm and a length adapted to the scar to be treated.

A marker film is taken to visualize the exact position of the Iridium 192 wire inside the needle. The reference isodose is at 2.5 mm from the axis of the wire, resulting in a cylindrical target volume, having the same length as the wire and a diameter of 5 mm. A dose of 1200 rads is delivered in about 8 to 16 hours depending upon the activity of the Iridium 192 wire (Figure 62). The removal of

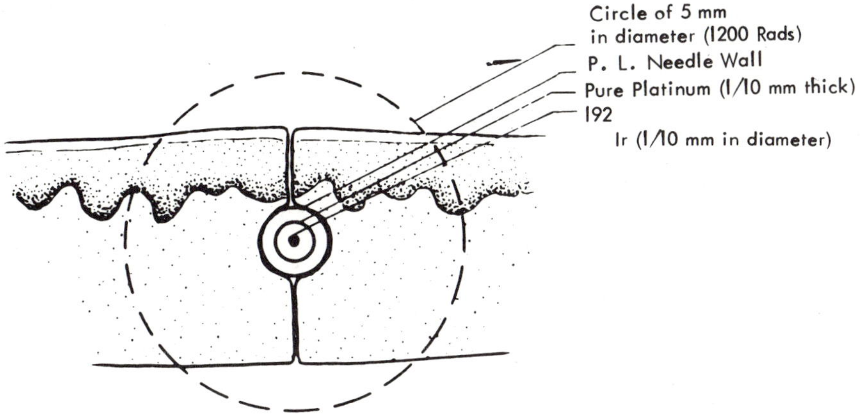

Figure 62. Keloids. Cross section of hypodermic needle technique.

the needle does not require any anesthetic, and there is usually no bleeding.

If the keloid is in proximity to radiosensitive organs such as the eye, growing cartilage in a child, gonads, etc., it is preferable to abstain from the use of endophoton therapy, and to consider teletherapy using well focused, low energy x rays, or to use electron therapy with Yttrium 90 needles.

C. Therapeutic Results: We have irradiated 13 patients with this technique, some of whom had multiple keloids totalling about 20 lesions. We have seen 3 cases of recurrence at the edges of the target volume which were due to technical errors, the Iridium 192 wire having failed to cover the entire length of the surgical scar. All other cases have been controlled, but not all of the results have been cosmetically good.

Localized Malignant Lesions

a. Clinical Anatomical Review: The majority of the malignant lesions of the skin are squamous cell or basal cell carcinomas. They are usually located on exposed areas of the skin; and more particularly on the upper half of the face, that is, the nose, frontal region, temporal regions, eyelids and the ears, which are more exposed to sunlight. They usually evolve from chronic dermatoses or dyskeratoses. In general, they grow rather slowly and offer excellent indications for endotherapy or plesiotherapy. Cutaneous metastases of various adenocarcinomas can be well treated with endotherapy, provided they are isolated lesions.

We will discuss the technical considerations relating to the thickness and extent of these lesions, and for several specific locations; namely, the nose and the ear. It is important to outline the edges of these lesions with a dermatographic pencil in order to establish an accurate target volume before starting any procedure.

b. Recommended Techniques: Superficial lesions less than 1 mm thick. This is usually the situation of dyskeratoses as well as for superficial carcinoma exemplified by the classical cicatricial carcinomas of the skin. We recommend plesioelectron therapy with P^{32} or Sr^{90} applicators. It is important to include a 4 to 5 mm margin of normal skin in the target volume. The dose should be about 10,000 rads per application, which requires a few hours with P^{32} or a few minutes with Sr^{90}. A very intense radioepidermitis becomes apparent in the days following, resulting in desquamation and healing in about 3 weeks. A second application of 10,000 rads at the surface of the epidermis results in the absorption of only 3500 rads at a depth of 1 mm for P^{32} and 4000 rads for Sr^{90}. The resultant scar is usually pale and slightly depressed, but quite soft.

For lesions which are minimally or moderately extensive, that is up to 4 cm in diameter, we recommend the hypodermic needle or silk suture technique (local or basal anesthesia). A wide margin of normal skin is included in the dose of 6500 to 7000 rads given at the reference isodose. The dosimetry is done either directly on a drawing from measurements taken on the skin, or from a tomogram (especially necessary when two planes of implantation are used).

Other Technical Modality
Silk Suture Technique

Modified from the original technique of SAHATCHIEV AND MOUCHMOV.

In this technique, a thin pliable silk suture carrying a length of radioactive wire is sewn directly into a lesion.

A #4 silk suture, about 100 cm in length, is prepared in the following manner:

At 10 cm from one of its ends, a hole is perforated in the wall of the suture with a rigid metallic wire 0.4 mm in diameter, which is then threaded upward inside the suture for a short distance. This portion of the silk suture is then dipped into a solution of resin of perchlorvinyl and 30% acetone. After the acetone has evaporated and the resin solidifies, the wire is removed, leaving a rigid cannula.

Iridium 192 wire of the desired length is introduced into the silk suture through the cannula thus formed. The silk suture is knotted at the distal end of the radioactive wire, to serve as a stop when the silk suture is pulled through tissues.

At the proximal end of the silk suture, a piece of adhesive tape is folded, on which the identification number of the wire is marked.

To insert the radioactive wire into a tumor, a surgical needle is threaded onto the proximal end of the silk suture, after removing the identification tape. The needle shape is selected which best fits the anatomical condition. One of the advantages of this technique, is the possibility of implanting curved surfaces.

The other advantage of this technique is the exceptionally good tolerance of the material during the implantation. This somewhat complicated, yet sophisticated technique is, therefore, recommended in certain situations, for example, for carcinomas of the inner canthus of the eye.

Lesions of the Nose

Carcinomas of the nose occur rather commonly. The complex architecture of the pyramid of the nose necessitates technical modalities adapted to its different structures. We will discuss four distinct locations on the nose, namely, the alae nasi, the dorsum of the nose, the septum and the bridge of the nose.

Ala Nasi: Whether these carcinomas have their origin on the mucosa, which is rather rare, or on the skin, as is most frequently the case, the technique best adapted to these lesions is either the hypodermic needle or the silk suture technique (basal or local anesthesia). The implantation is performed in a direction as parallel as possible to the border of the nostril, and overrides into the nasolabial junction, if the extension of the tumor requires it.

Dorsum of the Nose: We recommend the same general techniques. The usual extension of these lesions towards the ala nasi requires a slightly oblique orientation of the implant in relation to the main axis of the dorsum of the nose, in order to maintain a constant spacing between the radioactive sources, and to adequately irradiate the dorsum of the nose and the adjacent right or left side of the nose.

Nasal Septum: Whether the lesion has originated on the cutaneous or mucosal surface of the nasal septum, we recommend the guide gutter technique of endotherapy (basal or local anesthesia).

The implantation is achieved upward in the plane of the nasal septum. A single hairpin 2 to 3 cm long is usually sufficient to cover its entire width. If the lesion extends beyond the septum, it is possible to add one or two single radioactive sources, being careful to maintain a constant spacing between them. If necessary, one can also place a plastic mold in the affected nostril in order to separate the ala nasi from the nasal septum. The pins are then sutured at the inferior border of the nasal septum or nostril.

An alternative method of treating lesions of the nasal septum, is by the hypodermic needle technique, transfixing the nose and maintaining parallelism with plexiglass plaques.

Bridge of the Nose Including Naso-orbital Regions: When lesions extend beyond either side of the bridge of the nose, they approach the medial canthus of the eye. For small lesions of this region, we recommend using the silk suture technique, which is best adapted to the natural curvature of this region. For large lesions extending over the major portion of the nasal pyramid and often exceeding its margins, the plastic tube technique is preferable.

Lesions of the Eyelids

Most of these lesions are basal cell carcinomas arising from the margins of the lower eyelids. The silk suture technique is best for all tumors of the eyelid. Normally only a single radioactive line threaded very carefully just beneath the surface of the lid margin is necessary. The patient must be monitored closely during the application to be sure that this implant remains in place, since the eyelid tissues are quite fragile.

Lesions of the Ear

The indications for brachytherapy of carcinomas of the ear are for lesions involving the pinna or adjacent cutaneous structures. Lesions of the external auditory canal are best treated by surgical removal or by teletherapy, preferably with electrons.

Despite, and because of the complexity of the structures of the pinna of the ear, endotherapy is used in a relatively simple manner. Whatever the location of the carcinoma, it is preferable to simplify the implantation to a rectangular form with parallel lines anchored in healthy tissues, and if necessary suspended in free air to form bridges from one point to another. Thus endotherapy and plesiotherapy are used simultaneously in one target volume.

We recommend the hypodermic needle technique (basal or local anesthesia). These fine needles can easily penetrate the thin skin and cartilage of the ear. To anchor them adequately, it is often necessary to use much longer needles than are needed to cover the target volume. The orientation of the radioactive sources is variable, depending upon the location of the lesion, but the implantation should be in the vertical direction as much as possible. If necessary, the target volume is allowed to extend beyond the anatomical boundaries of the ear to allow an adequate margin of irradiation. For lesions of the retroauricular groove, it may be necessary to bring the ear closer to the mastoid region by suturing it, or to increase the spacing between these structures with dressings.

For superficial lesions of the helix, the silk suture technique using one or two radioactive lines may work best.

c. Therapeutic Results [4, 5, 6]: The therapeutic results are generally very satisfactory for superficial lesions. If a recurrence develops at the border of the treated area, an application of beta therapy can be made without risking necrosis, even if it overlaps the previous target volume.

The results of treating larger lesions with these new techniques needs to be carefully analyzed. We are impressed by the esthetic results, especially for small lesions less than 3 cm in diameter. In these a total reconstruction of the skin is noted and an almost perfect control rate is achieved.

Since 1961, we have treated 338 carcinomas of the skin. From this group, we can take the example of carcinomas of the nose, in which 52 of 55 cases have been cured; and the example of carcinomas of the ear in which 38 of 39 cases appear to be cured. These control rates are similar for all skin lesions. In a group of 12 T_4 lesions of the nose or ear treated with these techniques, only one residual tumor was described (Figures 63(a, b) 64(a, b)).

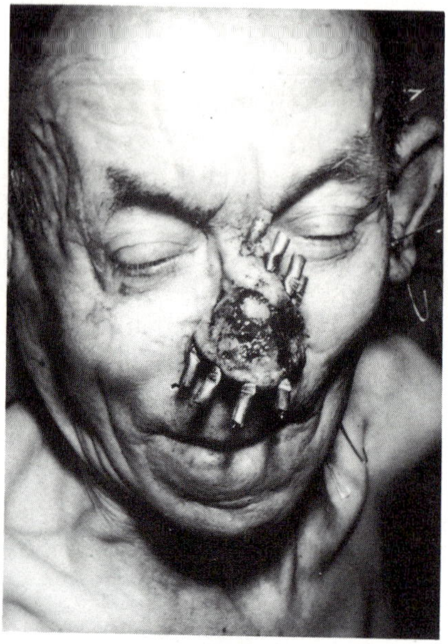

Figure 63. Squamous carcinoma dorsum of nose and ala nasi, locally advanced.

a. Hypodermic needle technique.

b. Same patient 1 year later.

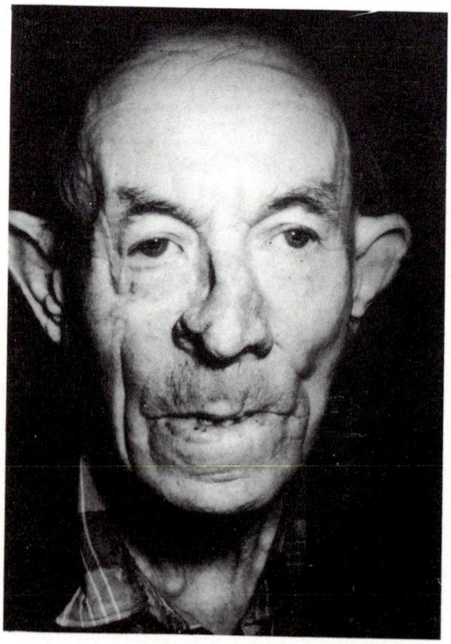

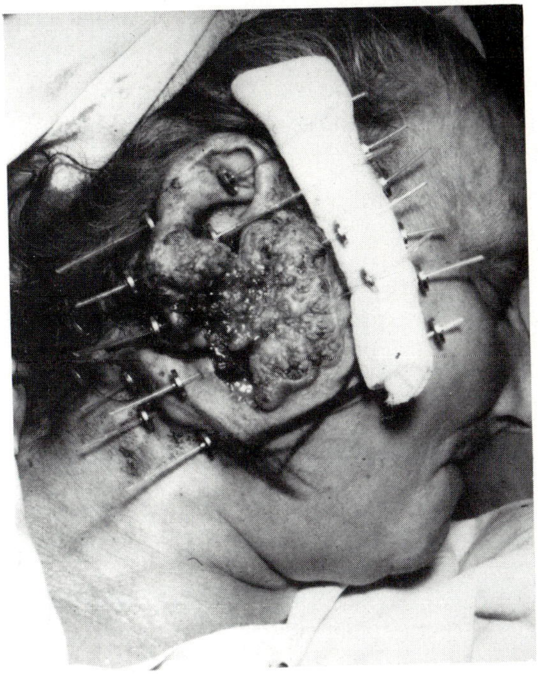

Figure 64. Squamous carcinoma, Right ear, locally advanced.
a. Plastic tube technique. 9 tubes in 2 planes.
b. Same patient 4 years later.

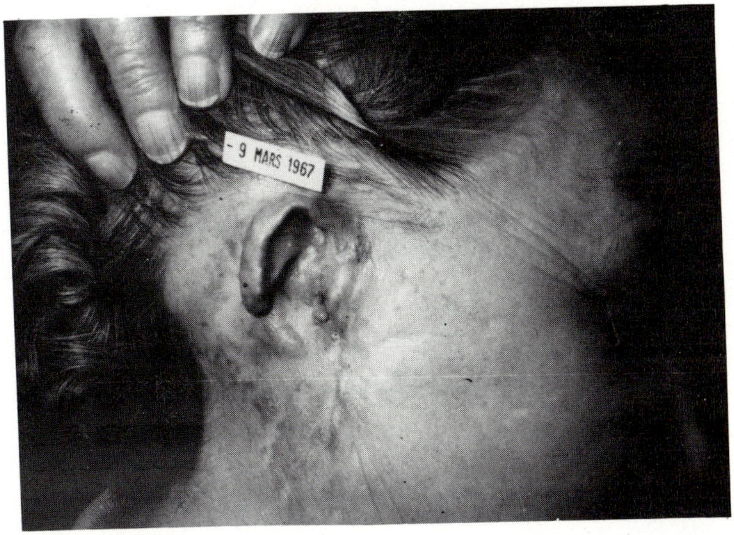

We conclude that the results of brachytherapy for carcinomas of the skin are excellent. The only restriction is for the more infiltrating lesions which invade the structures underlying the skin with the exception of the cartilages of the nose or the ear, which can be incorporated in the target volume without great risk of necrosis.

REFERENCES

1. Dana, M.: Applications en dérmatologie des téchniques modérnes en radio-thérapie, *Prèsse Médicale, 70:*1143-1145 et 1207-1208, 1962.
2. Nicoletis, C., et Chassagne, D,: L'irradiation intérstitielle par l'Iridium 192 dans la prévention des récidives après excision chirurgicale des cicatrices chet dlennes, *Annates de Chirugie Plastique, 2:*237-242, 1967.
3. Sahatchiev, A., Mouchmov, M.: "L'emploi des fils de soie radio-actifs dans la téchnique de brachyradiothérapie par tubes plastiques," 14:491-495, 1971.
4. Pierquin, B., Chassagne, D., De Maio, G., and Beyer, II.: "La radiothérapie des cancers épidérmoides de la peau par Iridium 192," *Annales de Radiologie, 12:*57-65, 1969.
5. Juillard , J. C.: "Apport de l'Iridium 192 dans le traitment des récidives des cancers cutanés de la face." Thèse pour le Doctorat en Médecine, Paris-Cretcil. 1971.
6. Pierquin, B., Chassagne, D., Cox, J. D.: "Toward consistent local control of certain malignant tumors." *Radiology, 99:*661-667, 1971.

Chapter IX

MALIGNANT NEOPLASMS OF THE FEMALE

Indications for brachytherapy are numerous in gynecology. This has been well established for carcinomas of the uterus where intracavitary plesiotherapy with radium has played an essential role since the early days of radiotherapy. This has not been true for carcinomas of the breast; except for some use of radium or Gold 198 endotherapy by Maisin surgery has had a dominant role until recently[1].

Our conviction is that brachytherapy can, and should share with surgery and teletherapy, an important role in the treatment of malignant tumors of the uterus and the breast. This development of indications for brachytherapy in gynecology is principally the result of new afterloading techniques which assure adequate protection of the medical personnel, despite the necessary use of numerous radioactive sources constituting a large quantity of radioactivity.

We will successively describe the use of brachytherapy in treating lesions of the breast, vagina, cervix and uterus.

THE BREAST

a. Clinical Anatomic Review: The breast is very accessible to endotherapy, despite its large surfaces and volumes and the problematic regional lymph node bearing areas. The brachytherapist is called upon to irradiate large target volumes, where the use of afterloading techniques is indispensable to provide adequate protection. We will discuss the indications for endotherapy in moderately extensive carcinomas of the breast, following tumorectomy or following external irradiation[2]. We will also discuss the use of brachytherapy in treating limited postoperative recurrences on the chest wall.

b. Recommended Technique: Small or moderately extensive carcinomas. In these cases, endotherapy is usually for delivering a "boost" dose following comprehensive external irradiation, with or without prior tumorectomy.

We recommend and describe in detail, the guide needle technique (basal or general anesthesia, patient supine).

This method is in reality a modification of the plastic tube technique adapted to the particular conditions of the mammary region. Tumors of the breast are usually situated in the midst of soft and movable tissues, where parallelism of radioactive sources cannot be adequately obtained, except by using rigid needles, which are themselves held in place at either end of the radioactive setup by plaques of plexiglass, which have been symmetrically perforated for the introduction of the needle. By referring to the original diagram and clinical description of the lesion, and to the mammograms and xerograms of the breast, the original boundaries of the tumor are drawn upon the skin of the breast, using a dermatographic pencil. Then the target volume is designated, systematically defining a large area of the breast to be included in the field of irradiation, generally constituting 25 to 30% of the total volume of the gland. The areolar region, which is a frequent site of microscopic extension, is always included. This target volume is oriented radially around the nipple.

After establishing the target volume, the exact point of entry and exit of each needle is marked, spacing them by 15 to 18 mm. Depending on the thickness of the mammary tissue, one or two planes of radioactive sources are used. If a second plane is necessary, its sources alternate with the sources of the first plane. It is important to leave a sufficient thickness of tissue between the radioactive sources and the chest wall on one side, and the surface of the skin on the other, to avoid creating areas of overdosage to either ribs or skin. (Figure 63ab).

The proposed spacing of the radioactive sources is then reproduced on plexiglass sheets 1 mm thick. The position of each radioactive line is indicated and two plaques of a convenient size are then cut from the sheets. Each point is perforated with heat to a diameter of 2 mm to allow easy transit of the guide needles, which are 1.6 mm in diameter. Finally, the edges of each plaque are padded with adhesive tape.

Implantation of the guide needles is then achieved. It is advisable that the implantation be performed, as much as possible, from the medial aspect. This facilitates the later afterloading, which is more safely and easily accomplished from the medial aspect, and allows removal of the dangerous needle points with cutting pliers. If two planes of implantation are necessary, the deeper plane is done first. When all of the needles have been implanted, the plexiglass plaques are sterilized in an antiseptic solution, slipped over the protruding ends of the needles and brought lightly into contact with the skin. Once these are in position, the immobilization buttons are slipped over the ends of each needle, and brought into contact with the external surfaces of the plaques. After adjusting the respective position of the plaques to produce the optimum target volume, the lateral immobilization buttons are crimped in place well in contact with the plexiglass, and the points of the needles on the lateral side are cut off a few mm beyond the buttons with wire cutting pliers.

By inserting a solid stainless steel obturator inside the guide needles, the medial immobilization buttons are crimped sufficiently to immobilize the plaque in position, yet not obliterate the lumen of the needle.

The exact required length of the radioactive sources is then measured, remembering to allow a few mm of unirradiated tissue at the entry and exit of the needles to avoid undue radiation effect on the skin (Figure 65 (a, b)).

Dosimetry can be achieved directly from a diagram taken from the plaques or preferably by obtaining a tomogram perpendicular to the plane of the implantation which offers the advantage of better establishing the relationship of the radioactive sources to the skin and ribs (Figure 65 (c, d, e)).

Finally, Iridium 192 wires are prepared in small plastic tubes, introduced into the medial ends of the guide needles and fixed in place with adhesive tape.

The dose calculated at the reference isodose depends on whether or not the brachytherapy has been preceeded by teletherapy. If 4500 rads have already been given with teletherapy, a boost dose of 4000 rads is added by the endotherapy. This boost dose is reduced to 2500 rads when the patient has had prior tumorectomy. If the total treatment is by endotherapy alone, approximately 7000 rads are given. Thus, when the patient has not had a tumorectomy, the total tumor dose is about 9000 to 10,000 rads, and a dose of not less than 8500 rads is distributed throughout the diseased quadrant. It is

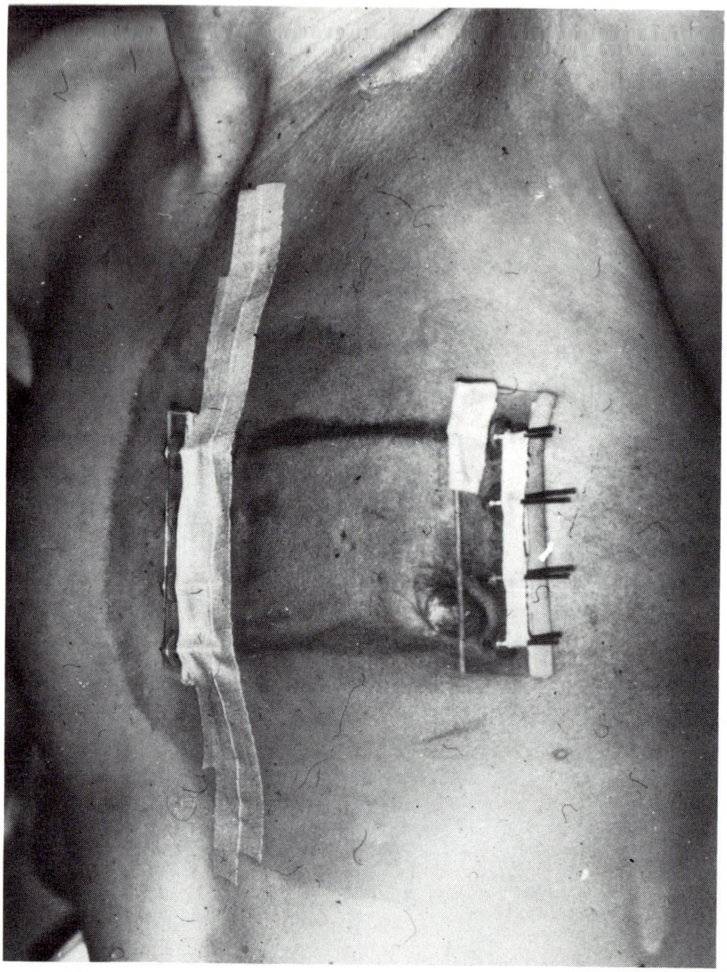

Figure 65. Cancer of the Breast. Guide Needle Technique of Implantation.

a. Single plane implant. 4 radioactive lines

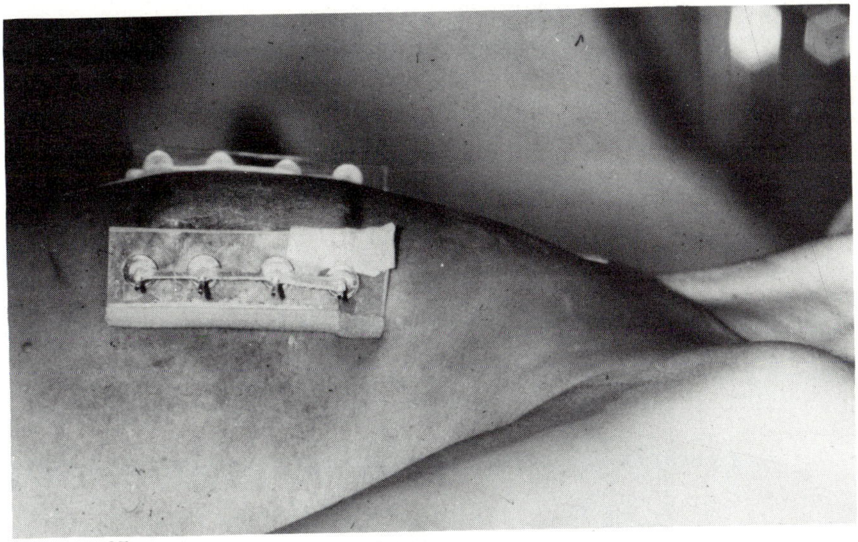

Figure 65.
b. Lateral view. Note lucite spacers and immobilization buttons in position.

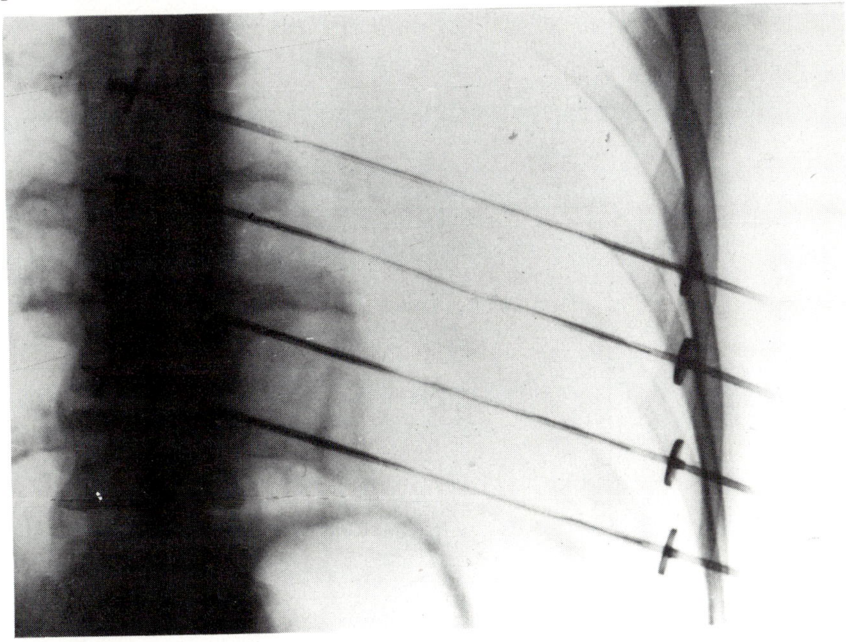

Figure 65.
c. Frontal roentgenogram. Guide needles have been after-loaded.

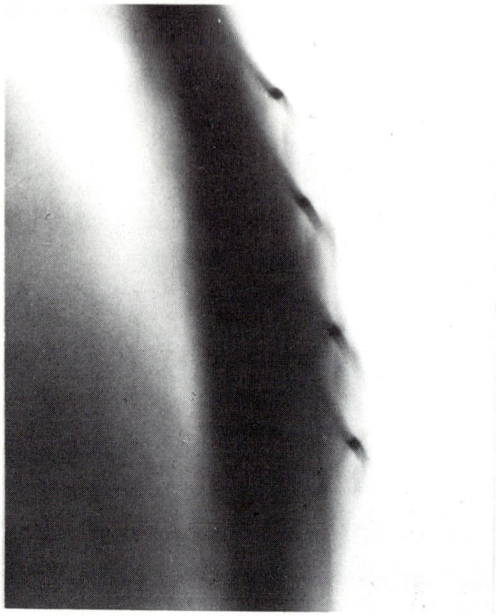

Figure 65.
d. Tomogram showing relationship of implant to chest wall structures.

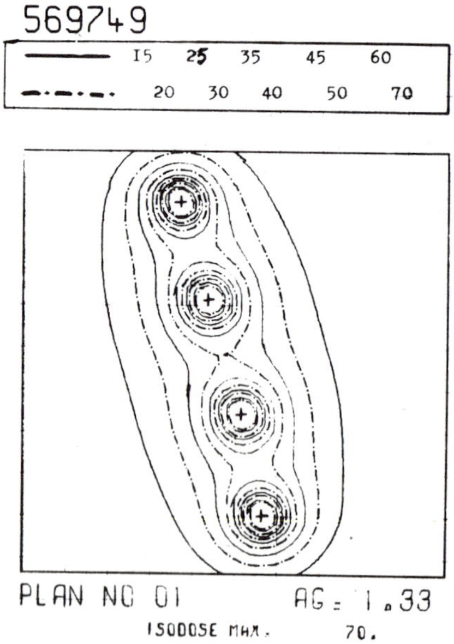

Figure 65.
e. Representative dosimetry. Reference isodose = 25 rad/hr.

estimated that the remainder of the breast tissue receives about 1000 rads.

The removal of this setup is very simple. After removing the radioactive sources, the needles are cut with pliers at the inner surface of the medial plaque. After smoothing the cut ends, to avoid traumatizing the tissues at the time of extraction, the entire setup is removed by pulling on the lateral plaque.

Limited Recurrences Following Surgery. The recurrences which are suitable for brachytherapy are usually located near the surgical scar. They are usually less than 1 cm thick, but fixed to the chest wall at depth. The diameter of the lesion usually does not exceed 5 cm.

We recommend endotherapy by the plastic tube technique generally accomplished under local anesthesia. The implantation is usually a single plane at the base of the tumor with the radioactive sources placed perpendicularly to the greatest diameter of the target volume.

c. Therapeutic Results. Between 1961 and 1975, we treated 320 cancers of the breast including 80 T_1, 170 T_2 and 70 T_3 lesions. There have been 16 local recurrences; two recurrences were of T_1 lesions, five T_2 lesions and nine of T_3 lesions. An actuarial calculation predicts an eventual recurrence figure of 6% in the T_1 and T_2 categories, increasing to 25% for the T_3 lesions. Presently, we recommend the use of this technique for T_1 and T_2 lesions only, with or without tumorectomy.

The aesthetic results are generally excellent in the T_1 category, good in T_2, and more often mediocre in the T_3. It is also for this reason that we have restricted the indication for treating T_3 lesions with this technique.

THE VAGINA

a. Clincal Anatomical Review: The vagina is an expandable conduit surrounded by levator muscles in its lower portion, separated from the rectum by the rectovaginal septum, and from the bladder by the vesicovaginal septum. The vagina lends itself easily to endotherapy and plesiotherapy. Primary squamous cell carcinomas are rare, but the vagina is often involved secondarily by tumors originating from the cervix, endometrium, vulva and urethra. Endotherapy is indicated for small superficial lesions and for larger infiltrating lesions. Plesiotherapy is primarily used for large lesions with minimal infiltration.

b. Recommended Technique: Small lesions of the lower one third: We recommend endocurietherapy by the guide gutter technique (general anesthesia, lithotomy position). A vaginal mold is made prior to the implantation according to the technique described in the section, Carcinoma of the Cervix. The later purpose of this mold is to help maintain the radioactive material in a stationary position, and to increase the distance between the implant and the opposite healthy vaginal wall.

After inserting a Foley catheter, the guide gutters are implanted upwards along an axis parallel to the vaginal canal. One finger checks the exact relationship of the points of the guide to the superior border of the tumor. When in place, the vaginal mold is gently placed in the vagina and the parallelism is checked radiographically. Radioactive pins are then substituted for the guide gutters and sutured in place. In difficult cases, it may be advisable to afterload the guide gutters and to leave them in place during the irradiation. In either case, guide gutters without plaques are used. The vaginal mold is normally maintained in place without additional support.

The dosimetry is based on transverse tomography of the implant or done by computer.

Large Superficial Lesions: We recommend a vaginal applicator technique of plesiotherapy using Iridium 192 (general anesthesia, lithotomy position).

A vaginal applicator is made as above, upon which the radiotherapist draws the tumor and the desired radioactive lines. Grooves are made along these lines into which are glued plastic guide tubes with sealed distal ends.

The applicator is then introduced into the vaginal canal and usually remains well in place without additional support, since its upper portion is normally somewhat expanded. Each guide tube is identified with a color index at its proximal end. A dressing is applied on the vulva through which these tubes protrude and immobilization buttons are passed over the plastic tubes until they come into contact with the dressing. Dosimetric control is accomplished using dummy wires, and either transverse tomograpy or frontal oblique tomography with the patient standing up.

After determining their proper length, the small inner plastic tubes containing Iridium 192 wires are afterloaded into the outer plastic tubes and maintained in position by crushing the immobilization buttons.

Large Infiltrating Lesions: We recommend the plastic tube technique of endotherapy (basal or general anesthesia, lithotomy position).

In most cases, these lesions arise from the anterior and lateral walls of the vagina. Involvement of the posterior wall is less common.

A vaginal mold is made on the day before the procedure as above.

Depending on the thickness of the tumor, one or two planes of radioactive sources are used. After inserting a Foley catheter, each guide needle is implanted upwards starting at the skin of the perineum near the vulva. With one finger in the vagina, the operator guides the needle upward until it makes its exit in the vaginal cavity at a point 1 cm above the superior border of the tumor. To accomplish this, the needle is inclined slightly towards the vaginal cavity, and counterpressure is applied on the vaginal mucosa with the finger. A plastic obturator is then introduced into the guide needle; and when it is visible in the vaginal cavity, it is gradually brought out through the introitus. After extracting the guide needle, the outer plastic tube can be introduced over the plastic obturator. Several loops are thus formed, their exact position in the tissue constantly controlled by the index finger in the vagina. At the end of the procedure, the plastic applicator is reinserted into the vagina.

If the tumor is more than 1 cm thick, this plane of endotherapy can be supplemented by a second plane of radioactive sources fixed at a desired depth in the applicator.

Transverse tomography is done with dummy sources in place for the dosimetry (Figure 66 (a, b, c, d)).

Therapeutic Results: In a study carried out in 1969, we treated 13 cases of primary carcinoma of the vagina or the urethra with these techniques of brachytherapy. Six patients were living and well at

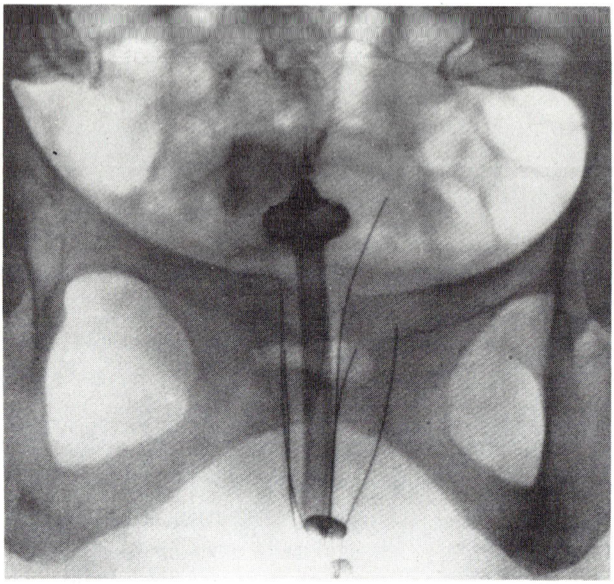

Figure 66. Carcinoma of the Vagina infiltrating the urethral meatus.
a. Endo-therapy via plastic tube technique. Frontal roentgenogram.

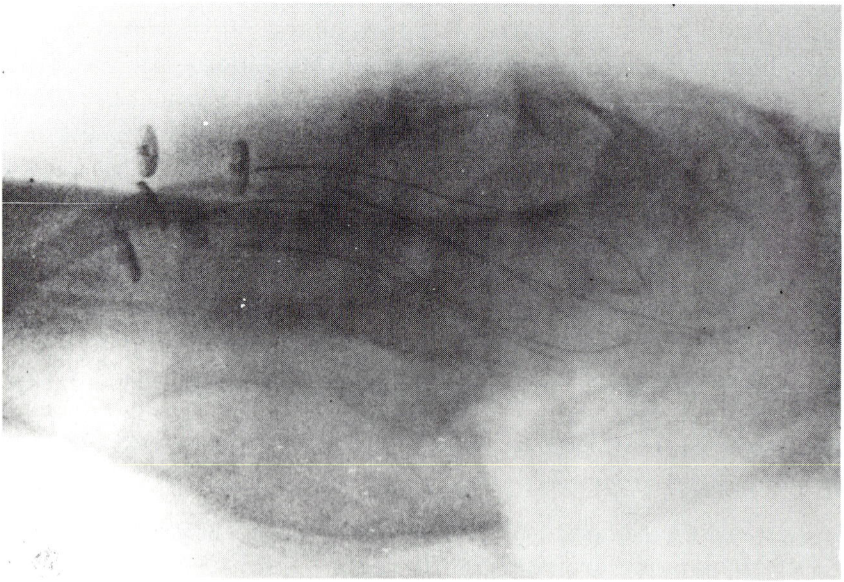

Figure 66. b. Lateral roentgenogram

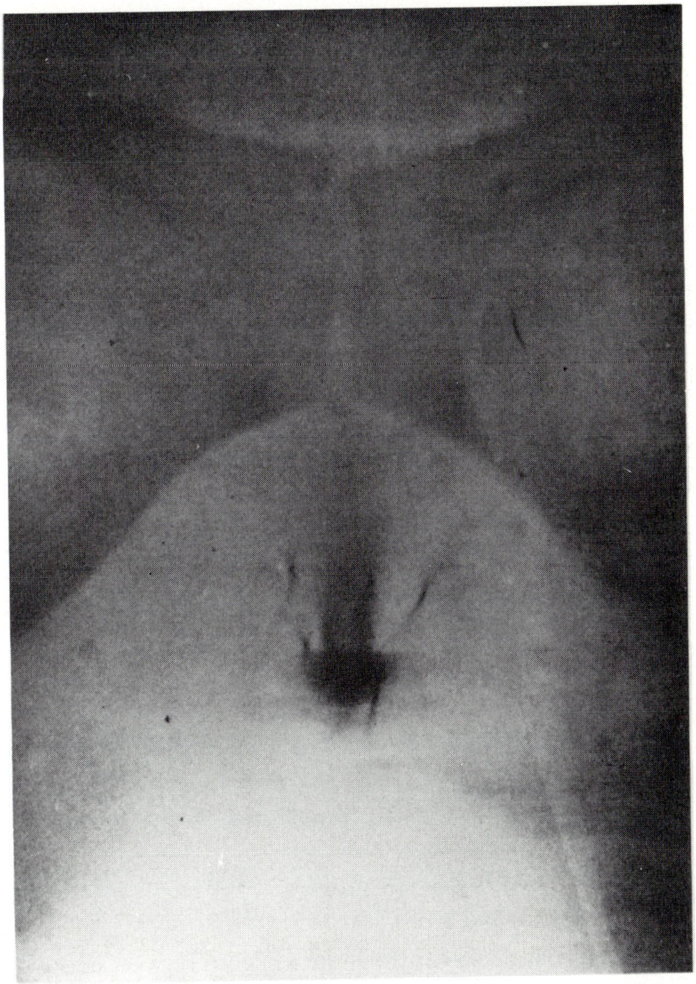

Figure 66.
c. Inclined frontal tomography.

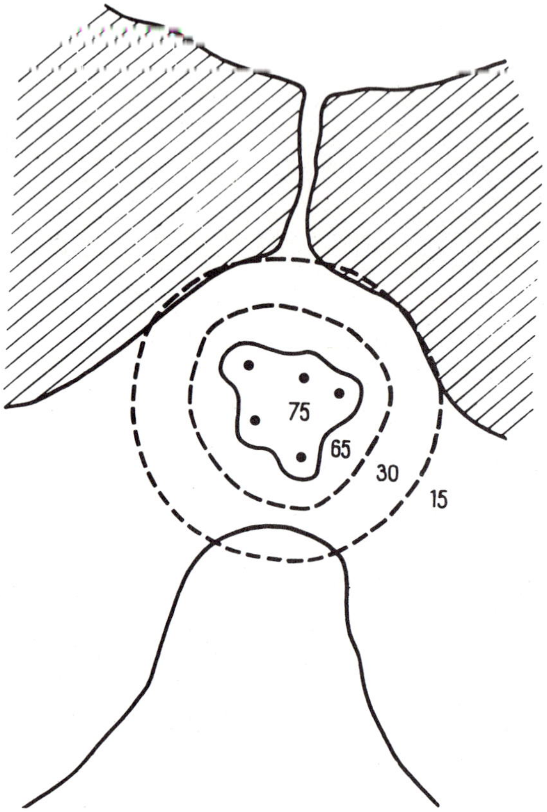

Figure 66. d. Diagram of dosimetry. 65 R/h per m Ci/cm at the reference isodose.

two years. There have been three local recurrences. Since 1969, we have treated 15 new cases with similar results.

THE CERVIX

a. Clinical Anatomical Review: Most cancers of the cervix are squamous cell carcinomas and uncommonly adenocarcinomas. The anatomical location of the cervix lends itself particularly well to plesiotherapy, for the cervix is surrounded by vaginal fornices which can accept large amounts of radioactive materials, and the cervix itself is perforated by the endocervical canal into which a radioactive catheter can be easily introduced. The cervix can, therefore, be irradiated with crossing beams of radiations emanating from endocavitary radioactive sources. This arrangement explains the favorable indications for curietherapy in the treatment of carcinoma of the cervix, and is the reason why techniques of radium plesiotherapy of the vagina and the uterus were the first to be so well established by Regaud and his staff at the Curie Foundation in the 1920's.

While irradiation of the cervix proper can be achieved under optimal conditions with plesiotherapy, it is less effective for some areas of possible tumor extension. Carcinoma of the cervix can extend upwards into the endocervical canal and endometrial cavity, laterally into the parametria and vaginal fornices and inferiorly along the vaginal walls. The bladder and rectum are invaded in late stages. For these peripheral structures, plesiotherapy cannot be satisfactory, because the dose decreases rapidly with distance from the radioactive material.

Plesiotherapy for the cervix is, therefore, used for rather early lesions of the cervix, either T_1 lesions strictly confined to the cervix itself, or T_2 lesions which extend only to the apex of the vagina or to the adjacent parametria. Beyond these limits, the use of plesiotherapy is only to compliment teletherapy. In the more extensive lesions (T_3 and T_4) and in special cases, some endotherapy techniques may be indicated.

We stress the excellent tolerance to ionizing radiations of the cervix, uterus and vaginal mucosa. The two immediately adjacent critical organs which tolerate radiations less well are the rectovaginal and vesicovaginal septum, which are, therefore, the limiting factor in this type of treatment.

b. Recommended Technique: We recommend a technique of plesiotherapy utilizing vaginal applicators afterloaded with either Cesium 137 seeds or Iridium 192 wires (basal anesthesia, lithotomy position).

This technique is based on four principles:

1. The precise adaptation of the technique to the individual lesion through the use of individually constructed vaginal mold applicators.

2. An accurate dosimetry based on a program of computer calcuations.

3. A nearly absolute protection of the medical and nonmedical personnel due to afterloading techniques and remote control projectors.

4. We insist upon the maintenance of a low-dose rate throughout the treatment and recommend maintaining the protraction of the Paris method.

VAGINAL MOLD APPLICATOR

Our experience with 1000 vaginal mold applications has shown that no two lesions are alike. In fact, there are numerous variables which change the anatomy in such a manner as to pose a particular problem in each case. These variables are:

—The size of the cervix which varies between 1 to 5 cm.
—The shape of the lips of the cervix.
—The position of the external cervical os.
—The apparent extent of the lesion and its thickness.
—The pliability and depth of the fornices.
—The dimensions of the vagina including its width, length and depth.

The anatomical variations are such that there is not one standard technique suitable for all cases. A vaginal mold applicator custom made for each case is perfectly adapted to both the lesion to be treated and to the individual anatomy.

FABRICATION OF THE VAGINAL MOLD APPLICATOR

A. Preparation of the Impression

The equipment consists of a 50 cc cake decorating syringe to which a rubber nozzle 3 cm long and 5 mm in diameter is attached, and an alginate powder, pink zelgan, which is commonly used for dental impressions.

With the patient in the lithotomy position and after washing the vulva and the vagina with antiseptic solution, one or two pieces of gauze, 15 cm long and 4 cm wide are introduced into the vagina. This gauze extends from the posterior fornix along the rectovaginal septum and protrudes from the vagina. The body of the syringe without plunger is then introduced into the vagina to the level of the labia minora. Gauze is wrapped around the syringe to obliterate the vaginal orifice.

An assistant quickly prepares the liquid paste by mixing equal parts of the alginate powder and cold water in a basin. This paste is then rapidly spooned into the body of the syringe, and then with a progressive and gentle pressure on the plunger, the vaginal canal is gradually filled with the alginate until it overflows and appears at the introitus of the vagina. To obtain a perfect mold, a constant pressure must be maintained.

The alginate solidifies in less than two minutes. The impression is then removed by asking the patient to bear down and by pulling on the gauze which became imbedded in the alginate (Figure 67).

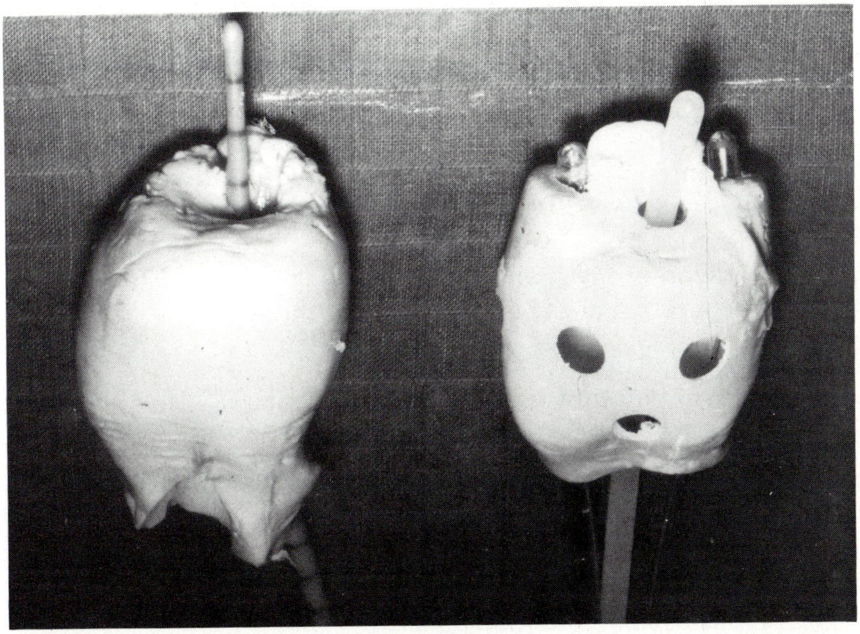

Figure 67. Cancer of the Cervix
Left: Alginate impression of the vagina. Note imprint of cervix tumor and urethra.
Right: Completed vaginal applicator. Uterine tube and plastic guide tubes have been positioned.

The general form of the vagina, as well as the location of the lesion and of the external os of the cervix, is easily identifiable on this impression. One may even sometimes detect a superficial extension of the tumor on the mucosa which was not visible by speculum examination and which could not be palpated. This mold constitutes a true 3 dimensional negative of the vaginal structures and of the tumor.

The portion of the impression which protruded outside the vagina is cut off with scissors. Generally, a ridge corresponding to the introitus of the vagina is visible and one can always find the imprint of the urethra on the anterior surface. On either side of the urethral imprint there are two small symmetrical elevations, which are essential to preserve. It is also advantageous to indent the proximal anterior surface of the mold to avoid compressing the urethral orifice later.

This impression is then covered with a wet pad to avoid its drying and shrinking.

The total time required for the preparation of this impression is about 5 minutes. The procedure should not be uncomfortable for the patient.

B. Preparation of the Applicator

The preparation of the applicator is in three steps:

1. Preparation of the Plaster Mold

In order to obtain a negative mold for making the applicator, about 300 cc of plaster of paris is prepared in a container in which the alginate impression is submerged. In one hour, the plaster solidifies, following which it is cut in two with a saw. The alginate impression is removed and the two halves of the plaster cast are rejoined.

2. Preparation of the Applicator

This plaster mold is painted with a thin film of obturator varnish (Stellon), which aids the subsequent removal of the applicator.

A synthetic autopolymerized resin (Pallavit) is prepared in a beaker by mixing the powder and its solvent until a thin paste is obtained. This paste is then poured into the plaster mold, while rotating it gently until the resin adheres to its walls and acquires a uniform thickness of about 2 to 3 mm. The paste solidifies completely within a few minutes and the two halves of the plaster mold can then be separated and the rough hollow applicator removed.

3. Preparation of the Applicator and Positioning of the Guides.

a) Position of the Radioactive Sources. This is the principle radiotherapeutic phase, whereby the number of radioactive sources, their spacing, their lengths and finally their depth, in relationship to the surface of the applicator are chosen.

At the site corresponding to the external os, an orifice, 8 mm in diameter is drilled. Symmetrical lateral radioactive sources are usually placed on either side of this orifice. Their length varies between 1 and 4 cm depending on the anteroposterior diameter of the cervix. Their spacing is a minimum of 15 mm and a maximum of 35 mm. If a spacing of more than 35 mm is to be considered, it is usually preferable to add a central third radioactive source near the orifice. This is usually in dealing with rather voluminous crevices, with large lateral fornices, in which it is not unusual to find a transverse diameter of the upper portion of the vagina exceeding 5 cm. Spacing and the depth are proportional to the length of the sources according to the following empirical table.

Length	*Spacing*	*Depth*
10 mm	15 mm	3 to 4 mm
20 mm	15 to 20 mm	4 to 5 mm
30 mm	20 to 30 mm	5 to 6 mm
40 mm	30 to 40 mm	5 to 6 mm

The best positioning of the vaginal sources is thus established and their location is traced on the exterior of the applicator with a pencil.

b) Insertion of the Guide Elements: Depending on the type of radioactive sources to be used, one chooses between inserting plastic tubes or incorporating such classical equipment as spheres, ovoids and corks. This work is achieved using dental drills of different caliber to modify the applicator. Small amounts of resin are used to glue the guide systems inside the applicator. It is sometimes necessary to reinforce some parts of the applicator by adding an additional layer of the synthetic resin. The entire duration of these procedures is about 30 minutes, depending on the experience of the operator.

c) Final Preparation: Polishing the applicator is necessary to avoid traumatizing the vaginal mucosa at the time of its insertion. It is also very useful to perforate several holes 3 to 4 mm in diameter on the different surfaces of the applicator. These holes have a triple purpose. They will make the applicator lighter, and once the applicator is positioned, the vaginal mucosa herniates through them, and this effect insures adequate immobilization of the applicator. Finally, they permit doing vaginal irrigation during the treatment via a soft multiply-perforated catheter, which is also fixed inside the hollow applicator with a dab of resin. (Figure 67)

I. Insertion of the Vaginal Applicator

Whenever possible, we prefer to perform the vaginal and uterine applications simultaneously.

1) One, therefore, proceeds in the usual manner with the patient under general anesthesia and in the lithotomy position. Following careful vulvovaginal antisepsis, a Foley catheter is inserted and the endocervical canal is dilated with Heggar dilators up to a number 7 or 8.

Following the dilatation, the length of the uterine cavity is accurately measured and the plastic intrauterine tube is introduced. The total length of this tube should be at least 30 cm so that it protrudes well beyond the vulva. The vaginal speculum is then removed, and the intrauterine tube is held in place by keeping slight pressure on it.

The vaginal applicator is then passed over the external portion of the intrauterine tube via the orifice drilled at the level of the cervical os. The free end of this tube is held while introducing the applicator into the vagina. The applicator is inserted at a 90° angle in relation to its final position, until it has been inserted three-fourths of the way into the vagina. It is then rotated back to the normal orientation. In order to be assured of the correct position, the two indentations on the anterior surface of the applicator should be in juxtaposition with the urethral region. The folds of the labia minora and labia majora should cover the edges of the applicator completely to avoid traumatizing the introitus.

The introduction is facilitated by adequately lubricating the introitus of the vagina and the surfaces of the applicator with surgical jelly. In addition, wooden tongue depressors introduced at the posterior vaginal fourchette to push the perineal region closer to the coccyx may be helpful.

All of these maneuvers are rather simple, provided constant pressure is maintained on the applicator during its insertion.

The uterine catheter is then attached to the vaginal applicator. The simplest technique is to use ordinary nylon sutures passed through the lower end of the posterior wall of the applicator, tying them around the uterine tube to form a semirigid connection between the applicator and the uterine tandem. To further secure the immobilization of the uterine tube, adhesive tape can be used. An alternative method is to glue the uterine tube to the applicator with more resin after checking the position of the applicator with marker films.

2) The vaginal applicator almost always maintains its desired position. During the first 24 hours, the patient is asked to remain at bed rest. Within a few hours, the vaginal mucosa herniates through the holes of the applicator, holding the latter firmly, and following which the patient is capable of sitting up in bed or of ambulating for a few minutes at a time during the day. She is, however, instructed to avoid putting any pressure on the abdomen, especially the efforts of having bowel movements.

The tolerance of this setup is astonishingly good during the 5 to 7 days of the application, because of the perfect anatomical fit and its light-weight, nonallergenic characteristics.

Daily vaginal irrigations eliminate all local infection and odor.

3) The insertion of the radioactive sources is different for Iridium 192 and Cesium 137, and will be discussed in detail at the end of this chapter.

The afterloading is, however, always preceeded by marker films taken with dummy sources with lengths equal to the ones planned for the radioactive sources. The marker films are taken on the operating table at the end of the insertion and before the patient wakes up. If the position of the sources is unsatisfactory, the setup is immediately corrected, and the final fixation of the intrauterine tube is done only after reviewing the films.

4) The removal of the radioactive sources, the vaginal applicator and the uterine tube can be accomplished simultaneously or in stages.

A short-lasting anesthesia facilitates the removal, although it is not necessary in the great majority of instances, so long as care is taken to free the herniated mucosa from the small holes and at the introitus with the finger before attempting to extract the applicator from the vaginal canal. The applicator should be turned 90° laterally before it is extracted gently downwards and anteriorly by pulling on its posterior inferior border with forceps.

II. Possible Errors in the Vaginal Applicator Technique

These errors are rather uncommon, but should be recognized since their prevention is quite possible.

A) A defective impression can be the result of a too liquid mixture of alginate, or contrarily of too rapid a solidification of the mixture, generally because the water was too warm. In both instances, the impression must be retaken.

B) Inability to extract the impression occurs in about one out of twenty cases and has numerous causes.

1) The patient refuses to push down, or the gauze has not been introduced deeply enough into the vagina or has been poorly positioned.

2) A very narrow introitus with a rather wide upper vagina. This is uncommon in patients with carcinoma of the cervix, but can occur in young nulliparous women.

3) A recent conization or amputation of the cervix which results in the alginate penetrating the endocervical canal, thus preventing its removal.

These difficulties may result in removing the impression in fragments, rendering it useless. The procedure should be repeated provided certain precautions are taken.

a. Two or three pieces of gauze are carefully placed in the posterior and both lateral fornices.

b. An anesthetic ointment is used on the vaginal walls and at the introitus.

c. A retractor is used to push the perineum towards the coccyx during the extraction.

d. If there is a gaping or recently operated cervical canal, a small piece of Vaseline gauze is placed inside the defect.

In our cases, we have never failed to successfully complete this technique.

C) Difficulties During the Preparation of the Applicator

1. We have already mentioned the shrinkage of the applicator due

to dessication. Keeping it covered with a wet pad usually solves this problem, and if the mold is to be prepared the following day, it is advisable that it be kept in a sealed plastic bag.

2. The plaster can break in several pieces, but it can easily be reconstituted with modelling clay, so that a satisfactory mold can still be prepared.

3. In cases of an incomplete or fragile applicator due to using too little resin, an additional layer of resin will correct the defect.

4. Incorrect positioning of the radioactive guides may result in a nonparallel setup; or the guides may be too superficially or too deeply located. These situations are almost always correctable, otherwise, one should not hesitate to repeat the procedure again.

D) Difficulties at the Time of the Insertion

1. In some multiparous women, the upper portion of the vagina distends excessively at the time of taking the impression. In these cases, it is advisable not to take a maximum impression under pressure, and practically, 100 cc of alginate should be the maximum amount utilized.

2. Displacement of the uterine tube while the applicator is being put in place is possible. It can accidentally slide out of the cervical canal or can be bent during the insertion of the applicator, and this is usually detected on the marker films. In these instances, one should reinsert the applicator making sure to hold the intrauterine tube at the desired level as the applicator slides over it. This difficulty is usually the consequence of a rather too narrow aperture in the end of the applicator which prevents it from sliding freely. The intrauterine tube should be made of a semirigid plastic material with a diameter of 6-7 mm. A rigid metallic tube, like that of the Fletcher-Suit applicator, could also be used.

3. Rather exceptionally, usually in elderly women with relaxed or shortened vaginas, the applicator may fall from the vagina during the treatment time. One may be obliged to use a T-shaped bandage applied to the inferior border of the applicator, or to suture the applicator to the lateral vaginal walls. In the latter event, the sutures should not be placed through the labia minora or majora, which can produce considerable discomfort, is inefficient and produces bothersome edema.

4. Vulvar or vaginal irritation or edema may result in some difficulty in the extraction of the applicator at the end of the treatment. This is the result of too long an applicator protruding beyond the introitus or to inadequate polishing of the edges of the applicator causing abrasions.

This enumeration of possible difficulties should not indicate that they are frequently encountered. They have been described in order to explain their causes, which are invariably due to faulty technique which can be prevented or corrected.

III. Protection of the Medical, Technical and Nursing Personnel

This vaginal applicator technique could certainly be used without afterloading. There is, however, no major advantage over other methods, unless the afterloading technique is used to protect the personnel. Two different types of radioactive sources are used.

The first type is rather simple, making use of Iridium 192 wires and the second is more elaborate, using Cesium 137 microspheres.

A. Iridium 192 Wires

We use Iridium 192 wires 0.5 mm in diameter with a linear activity of 5 to 7 mCi/cm for applications of 5 to 7 days. If the linear activity is less than 7 mCi/cm, the time of irradiation becomes considerably longer, although the wires are still useful for giving boost doses, such as in stage III lesions. When the activity drops below 5 mCi/cm, one can double the wires to produce the desired strength. In essence, 50 cm of Iridium 192 wire with a linear activity of 10 mCi/cm is sufficient for the treatment of three cases per week for three months.

As with the technique of endotherapy with plastic tubes, these wires are loaded into "inner" plastic tubes of a diameter adapted to the wires.

These tubes carrying the radioactive sources are then introduced into the "external" tubes that are incorporated into the applciator. These external tubes normally have a minimum external diameter of 3 mm and a maximum diameter of 6 mm. Our preference is the larger tubes 6 mm in diameter, of a semirigid consistency, especially for the intrauterine tube. Smaller sized tubes are acceptable for the lateral sources, and are occasionally indispensible in particularly curved or small applicators. In this respect, Iridium 192 wires are advantageous since they are quite malleable and can be introduced into markedly curved outer tubes.

The insertion of the radioactive sources is always preceeded by marker films. While the length of the vaginal sources can be established in advance, at the time of the preparation of the vaginal applicator, this is not the case for the length of the intrauterine source which is determined only after the setup has been inserted and marker films taken (Figure 68 (a, b)).

Insertion of the radioactive sources is done in the patient's room from behind a lead screen. The sources are fixed in place either with adhesive tape, by gluing the tubes with a small amount of synthetic resin, or by placing a tight cork in the external tube.

This manual afterloading method offers the advantage of simplicity. It also allows the periodic removal of the radioactive sources when the patient receives visitors or for nursing purposes, and can be reinserted in a few seconds.

The conditions of protection can be improved, however, with the use of a remote control projector to be described.

B. Cesium 137 Microsources

1. Description of the Sources

Cesium 137 was chosen because of its long half life and absent of risk of contamination.

These sources are commercially available in the form of seeds (see chapter III, Radioactive Material). Each seed of Cesium 137 is 3.5 mm long and 1.5 mm in diameter (Figure 3 (a, b)).

The maximum possible radioactivity in each seed is 25 mCi, but in practice, seeds containing 8 to 12 mCi or even less are used, since as many seeds as necessary can be added.

2. Description of the Cesium 137 Seed Holder

The seeds can be aligned with or without spacers in a pliable stainless steel springloaded tube with an internal diameter of 2 mm and an external diameter of 3.2 mm. These sourceholders are pre-assembled using a sequence of sources and inactive spacers to give the different desired active lengths. For routine purposes. sourceholders with an active length between 8 and 88 mm are used available in 8 mm intervals of length.

Dosimetric studies made by Dutreix and Wambersie[6] have shown that each such train of sources is equivalent to a continuous

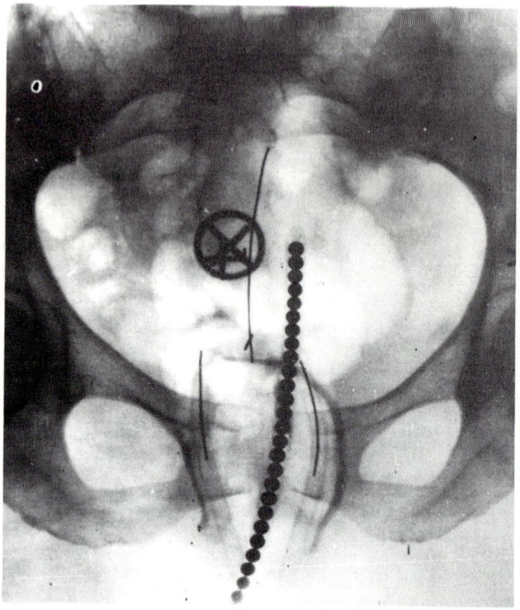

Figure 68. Cancer of the Cervix. Roentgenograms taken with I^{192} sources in position. Rectum identified by chain of lead beads.

a. Frontal view

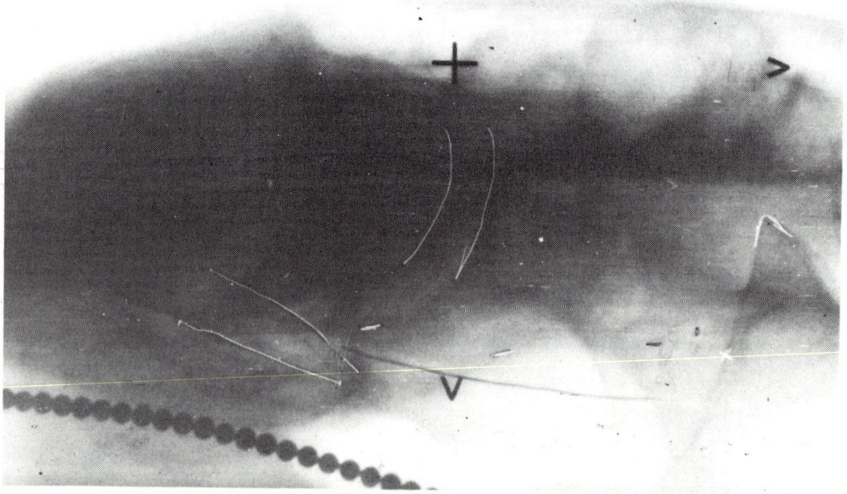

Figure 68. b. Lateral view

radioactive source of a length equal to the distance between the center of each end seen, plus one interval between the center of two adjacent seeds. For marker films, lead wires with a length equivalent to the length of each train of sources is used. These flexible holders can be introduced into the plastic tubes manually, however, they have been specifically manufactured for use with a remote afterloading projector, the Curietron (CGR MeV)[7].

Description of the Curietron

This unit consists of a remote control system which can inject or retract the sources in a few seconds. It rests on a four-wheeled cart which can be moved close to the patient's bed and connected to the patient by means of flexible lightweight ejection sleeves.

In the resting, nonirradiation mode, the sources remain in a shielded box with a total radioactive capacity of 300 mCi, yielding a dose on its surface not exceeding 2.5 mr/hr.

Four sourceholders can be ejected simultaneously. They are equipped with individual electromagnetic systems with a moving cable to push the sources out of the shielded box through the transfer sleeves into the external tubes placed in the patient.

An electric safety device assures the satisfactory position of each source in the external tubes. A record of the total exposure time is automatically made by four independent counters. In addition, numerous other safety devices are also added including a safety key, a low-voltage circuitry and a manual system for the return of the sources to the safety box in the event of an electrical failure (Figure 69).

In routine use, the Curietron carries three source ejectors, namely, the two vaginal and the single uterine sources. After marker films have been taken, the patient is returned to her bed. Usually, one to two hours are allowed before connecting the end of each plastic tube to the ejection sleeves. In the storage room, sourceholders of desired active lengths are transferred to the Curietron by remote control.

Once the connection is made, it is indispensable to attach the ejection sleeves to a metallic crib suspended over the patient's feet. The patient can then move easily in her bed (Figure 70).

With the remote control system placed outside of the patient's room, one can insert the sources, or return them to the Curietron each time the patient's room is entered for nursing care or for visits.

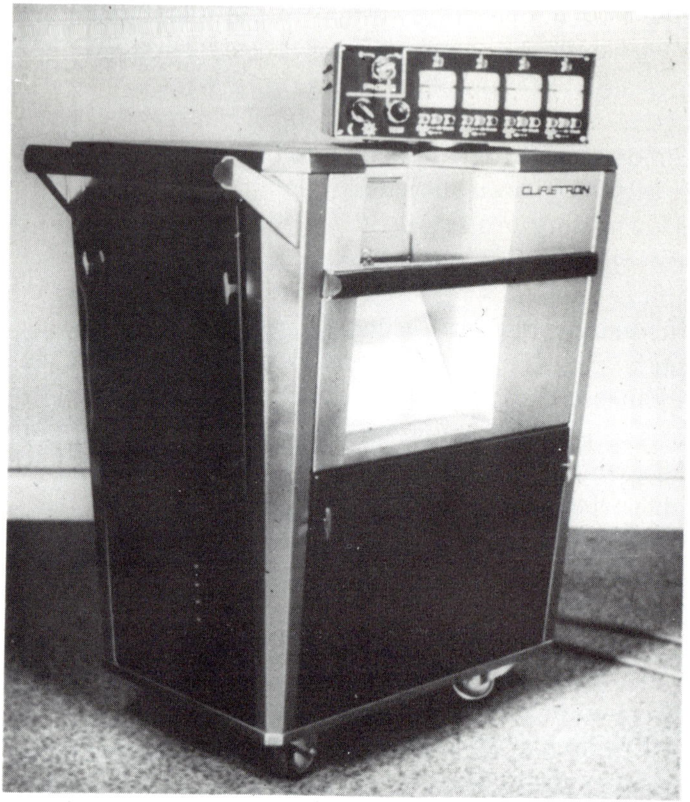

Figure 69. Remote afterloader. The Curietron.

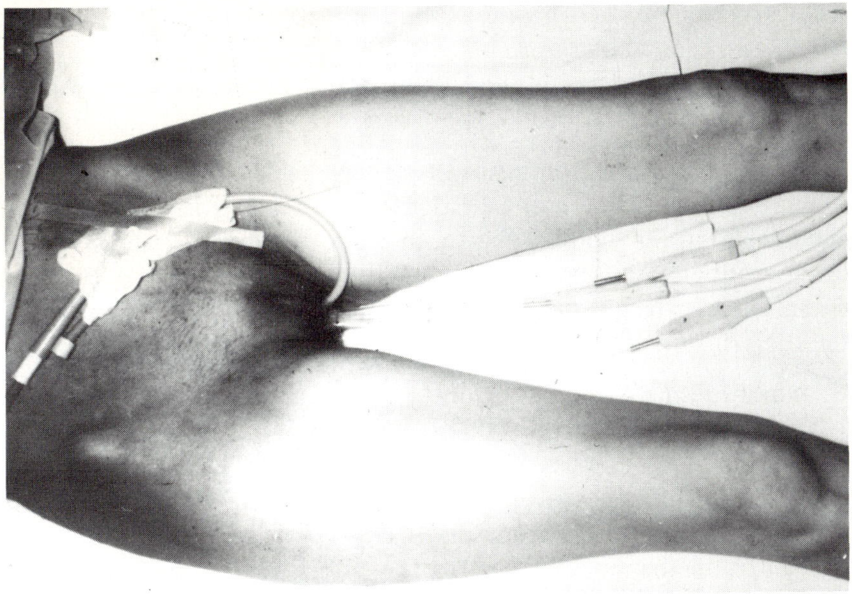

Figure 70. Cancer of the Cervix.
The vaginal applicator has been inserted into the vagina and is connected to the ejection sleeves of the remote afterloader.

In addition, the ejection sleeves are disconnected from the external tubes for approximately one hour each morning to allow the patient to ambulate.

On an average, an interruption of one to two hours per 24 hours is accounted for during the calculation of the total time of irradiation. With this system, all radiation exposure to the hospital personnel is eliminated. The cooperation of the patient is usually excellent, and she actively participates in her treatment.

IV. Computer Dosimetry

Since January, 1968, a computer program has been perfected by A. Dutreix and J. Rosenwald at the Institut Gustave Roussy and at the Foundation Curie [8].

Computer dosimetry is the third essential prerequisite for these gynecological techniques.

A. Functions of the Computer Program

The absorbed dose can be calculated at any point, taking into consideration the isotope, the tissue attentuation and the filtration by the envelopes, but without taking into account the oblique filtration and the auto-absorption of the sources, which is negligible for the Iridium 192 wires and the Cesium 137 microsources.

B. Marker Films and Study Data

Two marker films are taken in a strictly orthogonal position, made possible by using a special cassette holder. The position of each radioactive source is established by the coordinates of its two ends in a three dimensional system in relation to bony landmarks and, therefore, to the patient, and to the plane of the two films, and, therefore, of the cassette holder.

In addition, the following landmarks are routinely identified.

1. The anterior and posterior lips of the cervix and any other points of interest in the vicinity of the lesion, such as the lower limit of any vaginal extension, using silver clips implanted at a 1 cm depth according to the Delclos technique [9]

2. The rectum is outlined with a soft rectal catheter containing lead beads.

3. The region of the trigone of the bladder is identified with 7 cc of radiopaque material injected into the balloon of the Foley catheter.

4. Each pelvic wall is defined by the intersection of three lines:

a. A horizontal line traced on the AP film passing tangentially along the superior margin of the two acetabula.

b. A vertical line traced on the AP film passing tangentially to the medial aspect of the acetabulum.

c. A line drawn on the lateral film joining the highest portion of the two acetabulae in a craniocaudad direction and a lateral projection of the pelvic point located at mid distance from these points.

Our treatment plan aims to deliver a dose of 6000 rads at the level of the external iliac chain of lymph nodes. We, therefore, add the dose delivered by the external irradiation and the dose delivered by brachytherapy, knowing very well that this addition is radiobiologically uninterpretable, in view of the marked difference in the dose rate with the two radiotherapeutic modes.

To avoid complications, this total dose seems to be quite satisfactory. In a few particular cases, we have allowed a maximum dose of 6500 rads to one side of the pelvis.

b. Dose at the Level of the Pelvic Wall: The points on the pelvic wall defined earlier are spaced by 10 to 11 cm, without being related to the position of the cervix, but instead to the bony pelvis.

Actually these points are situated more posteriorly and medially than the points of origin of the external iliac chain of lymph nodes, and, therefore, receive a dose 10% to 20% higher than that delivered to the external iliac lymph nodes.

These points are also used for the calculation of the dose to be delivered by external irradiation, since they almost always are situated at the level of the maximum dose.

In summary, we recommend curietherapy for carcinomas of the cervix, stage I and II, with a single application of about 6 days duration using the described technique. With a calculation of the dose at the points mentioned above, one obtains a true "brachytherapy identity card" for each case, which defines and characterizes each application much better than the expression of a single dose at one point.

SPECIAL CASES

1. In advanced stage II, stage III and even in certain bulky stage I lesions, we recommend the same brachytherapy technique following external irradiation. The duration of the brachytherapy is adjusted depending on the dose delivered by external irradiation. For instance, when the pelvis has received 5000 rads with external irradiation, the brachytherapy application has a duration of between 36 and 50 hours. The treated volume will receive a dose of at least 1000 rads, but the total dose to the rectum and bladder should not exceed 7500 rads as already stated.

2. In the case of a small or narrow vagina, at the upper portion, we recommend the vaginal mold technique with the uterine tube

protruding within the applicator, which replaces the usual vaginal source (protruding source). One should remember, however, that this technique is undersirable, and that the rectal dose is always high, with a significant risk of proctitis.

3. For carcinomas of the cervical stump, external irradiation is the main therapy, although when the cervix can still be sounded to a length of 1 to 2 cm, it is possible to give brachytherapy by inserting a central source in the canal of the cervical stump. In these cases, the treated volume is smaller than when the uterus is intact.

c. *Therapeutic Results*

Our technique of treatment with Cesium 137, vaginal mold applicators and computer dosimetry has been well systematized only since 1970. We, therefore, lack a sufficient followup; nevertheless, the first results from the years 1969 and '70 indicate a survival at 5 years of 85% in stage I, 65% in stage II, 40% in stage III.

THE UTERINE CORPUS

A. Clinical Anatomical Review: Carcinomas of the uterus are more common than those of the cervix. These are lesions located above the internal os, and more often occur in middle aged, post menopausal women. They remain within the confines of the uterus for a long time, and are almost always adenocarcinomas. We do not recommend any form of irradiation as a primary form of therapy. Surgery is the treatment of choice in these tumors which are easy to extirpate.

These tumors, however, may extend to the cervix or to the vaginal walls, making their total removal by surgery difficult, with a high percentage of recurrence at the level of the vaginal vault. To avoid the latter possibility, we recommend irradiating the apex of the vagina with preoperative plesiotherapy.

B. Recommended Technique: We recommend preoperative vaginal plesiotherapy with Cesium 137 or Iridium 192 via the afterloading technique. This application is not different than that used for carcinomas of the cervix, except that the intrauterine catheter is not indispensible. Intrauterine plesiocurietherapy is justifiable in inoperable cases.

In cases where surgery is contraindicated, we recommend a course of teletherapy to the entire pelvis followed by plesiotherapy similar to the technique for carcinoma of the cervix. An afterloading technique for packing the entire uterine cavity is currently under development for use in inoperable T_1 lesions.

REFERENCES

1. Maisin, J., Maisin, H., Keusters, J., Maisin, A. and de Cock, A.: Le traitement des cancers du sein opérables par curiepuncture ou implantation d'Au 198, *Journal de Radiologie, 52:*237-244, 1971.
2. Pierquin, B. Raynal, M., Chassagne, D., and Baillet, F.: Radiothérapie seule dans le traitment des cancers du sein. Expérience de Créteil, *Thérapeutiques non mutilantes des Cancéreuses du Sein.* 233-236. 1973, MASSON et Cie Publish. PARIS.
3. Calle, R., Fletcher G. H., Pierquin, B: Les bases de la radiothérapie curative des epitheliomas mammaires, *Journal de Radiologie, 54:*:929-938, 1973.
4. Chassagne, D., Attaia, A., Pierquin, B.: Résultats de l'endocuriethérapie par fils d'Iridium 192 en gynécologie, *Journal de Radiologie, 51:*223-228, 1970.
5. Pierquin, B: Particularités téchniques de la plésiocuriethérapie utérovaginale par iridium 192, *Journal de Radiol, 54:*959-962, 1973.
6. Dutreix A., Wambersie, A.: Etude de la répartition des doses autour de sources ponctuelles alignées, *Acta Radiol., 7:*389-400, 1958.
7. Chassagne, D., Delouche, G., Rocoplan, J. A., Piérquin, B., and Gest, J.: Description et premiers éssais du Curietron, *Journal de Radiologie, 50:*910-913, 1969.
8. Rosenwald, J.C., Dutreix, A.: Etude d'um programme sur ordinateur pour le calcul des doses en curiethérapie gynécologique, *Journal de Radiol., 51:*651-654, 1970.

Chapter X

GENITOURINARY SYSTEM

The indications for brachytherapy in the genitourinary system are of major or minor importance depending on the organ considered. For the penis and the penile urethra, the indications are dominant and exclusive. For the female urethra, they are equally dominant, while for the prostate gland and for the prostatic urethra, they are very limited. In the case of the urinary bladder, there are important indications, but only in close association with surgery.

PENIS

a. Clinical Anatomical Review: These are all epidermoid carcinomas. The lesion may be localized to the glans penis, occasionally at the level of the corona, but more often at the neck of the penis, underlying the prepuce.

b. Recommended Technique: We recommend the hypodermic needle technique of endotherapy following circumcision (supine position, general anesthesia) (Figure 72).

1. Under general anesthesia, a Foley catheter is first inserted.

2. Depending upon the extent of the tumor, an appropriate number of hypodermic needles are successively implanted in a plane perpendicular to the penile shaft. For a rather superficial lesion, a single plane of 2 or 3 radioactive sources may well be sufficient. For more infiltrating lesions, two planes are usually needed, one on either side of the urethra. Four sources may be sufficient to cover the entire glans, or six may be necessary if the lesion extends towards the corpora cavernosum. In essence the adaptation of the technique should be as precise as possible, depending on the clinical manifestations.

The length of each hypodermic needle depends on the thickness of tissue to be implanted, allowing a margin for the plexiglass plaque, and the necessary margin for blocking the hypodermic needle. This implies lengths varying between 4 and 6 cm.

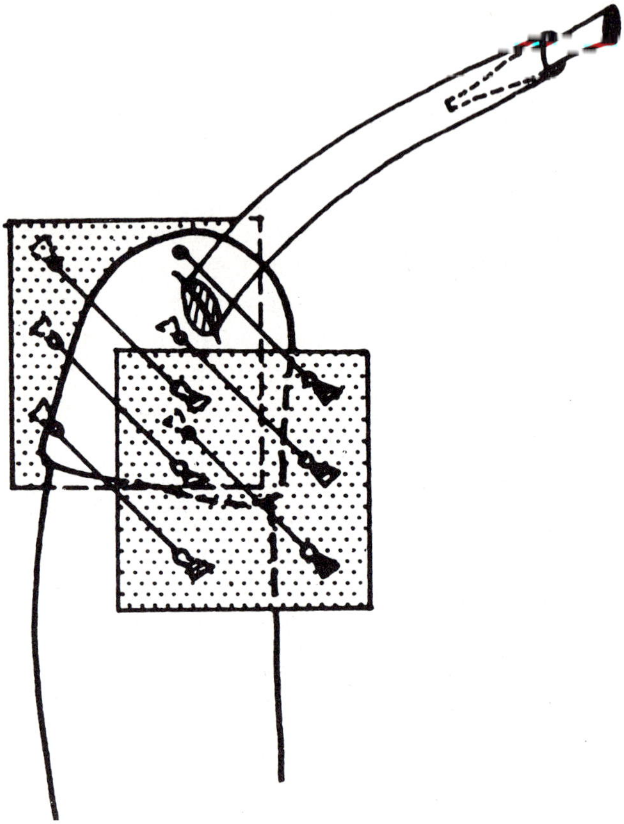

Figure 72. Cancer of the penis.
Hypodermic needle technique. 2 plane implant of 6 radioactive sources for a lesion of the glans penis.

3. Initially the needles are inserted in a random order, but their final position is corrected to insure perfect parallelism. The spacing between them is also kept quite uniform, and once it appears to be satisfactory, a drawing of the setup is made on a sheet of paper.

4. Plexiglass plaques 2 mm thick are cut and the position of each needle is marked on them. A hole corresponding to each needle is then perforated with heat. Finally, the edges of the plaques are covered with adhesive tape, and at the completion of the preparation they are immersed in an antiseptic solution.

5. The operator passes the two plaques over the ends of the hypodermic needles until they are in contact with either side of the penis, leaving the latter sandwiched between them.

6. The parallelism and the fixation of the two plaques is maintained by small pieces of adhesive tape at their upper and lower ends.

7. Lead buttons are then crimped on one end of each needle at the external surface of the corresponding plaque (Figure 73).

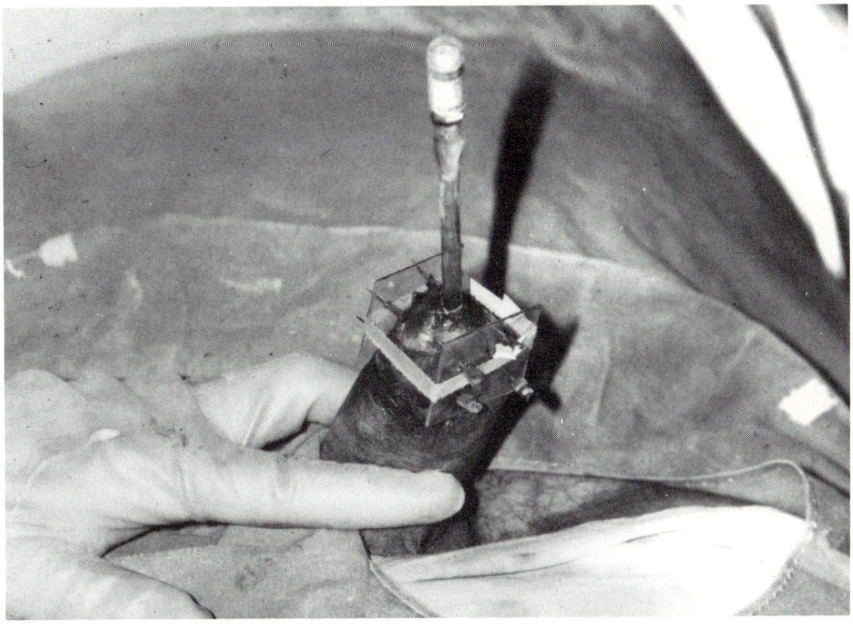

Figure 73. Cancer of the Penis.
Lead buttons have been crimped on the ends of the needles external to the lucite plaque.

8. When the non-radioactive preparation has been completed, the Iridium 192 wires are introduced, their length determined by the target volume to be irridated. Each wire is introduced from the open end of the corresponding hypodermic needle onto which a lead button is then crimped. This operation is performed from behind lead screen using long forceps.

9. During the treatment, the penis is maintained in a vertical position with the use of foam rubber, which keeps the radioactive setup away from the testes and the inner surface of the thighs.

10. The dosimetry is established by the Paris technique of "points", following the perforation of the plaque[1, 2]. 6000 rads are delivered on a reference isodose.

During the irradiation, which is usually between 4 and 6 days, the patient remains in bed, although he can ambulate occasionally.

In the days following this application, a severe radioepidermitis and radioepithelitis develop, associated with dysuria. These reactions subside in three weeks and scarring becomes evident between six and eight weeks.

c. Results: Between 1966 and 1971, we treated 45 carcinomas of the penis. These included 14 T_1 and T_2 lesions, 24 T_3a and 7 T_3b or T_4 lesions. In the T_1 and T_2 lesions, there have been only two local recurrences. In the T_3a group, there have been four local recurrences and one necrosis. In the T_3b and T_4 group, there have been four local recurrences and two necroses. It is concluded that this technique of brachytherapy is highly recommended for lesions that do not extend beyond the glans. For lesions that invade the corpora cavernosa or exceed 4 cm in diameter, surgery is preferred (Figure 74 (a, b)).

URETHRA

a. Clinical Anatomical Review: In males, it is important to distinguish between the penile urethra and the prostatic urethra. For the female urethra, it is equally important to remember that the therapeutic indications are similar to the vulva and vagina.

b. Recommended Technique: Penile Urethra: We recommend the hypodermic needle technique of endotherapy (supine position, general anesthesia).

Whether these lesions are primary carcinomas of the urethra or an extension of a carcinoma of the glans penis to the urethra, the technique of brachytherapy is identical to the one described for the penis. The radioactive implant, however, closely encompasses the tumor bearing area on both sides of the urethral canal.

Prostatic Urethra: We do not recommend brachytherapy for this portion of the male urethra (see prostate).

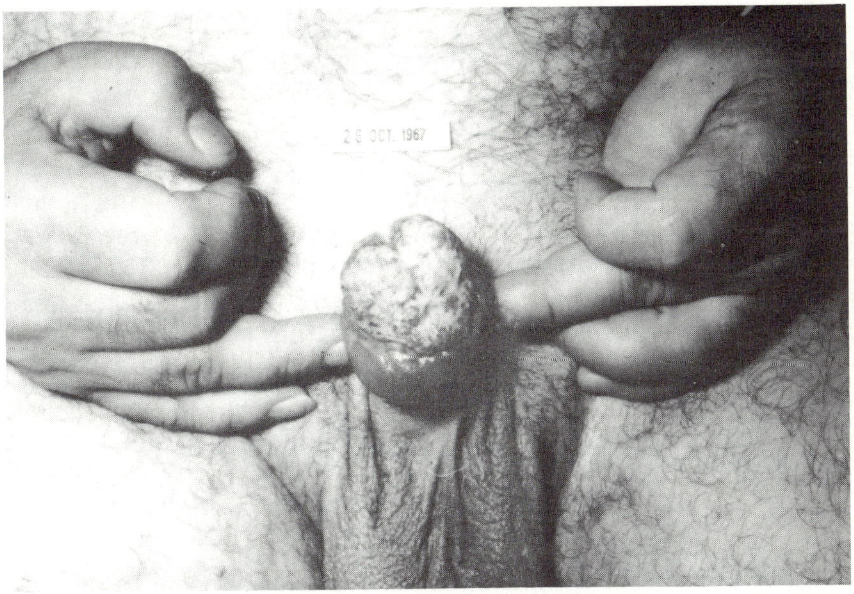

Figure 74. Cancer of the Penis

a. Extensive lesion of the glans penis treated by the hypodermic needle technique.

b. Local result 22 months post treatment.

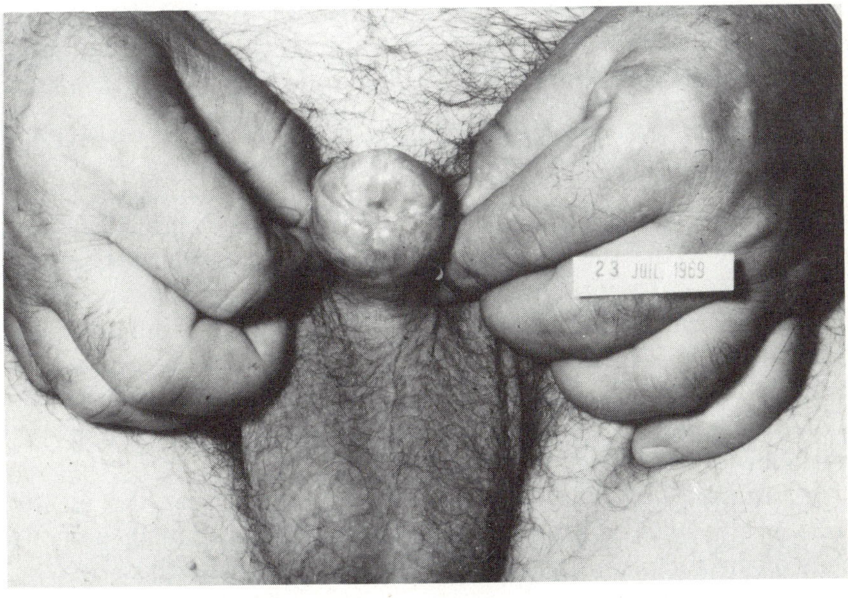

Female Urethra: In superficial lesions often surrounding the meatus, we recommend the guide gutter technique of endotherapy (lithotomy position, basal or local anesthesia).

After inserting a Foley catheter, the urethra is encompassed by two double guide gutters without lips which are implanted on either side of the urethral meatus, following a left and right sagital plane, and spaced according to the necessary dimensions of the target volume. The length of these guides is usually between 2 and 3 cm depending on the size of the lesion. If a length of 3 cm is exceeded, the radioactive material may risk penetrating the bladder.

Infiltrating lesions of the urethrovaginal region are treated in the same manner as infiltrating carcinomas of the vagina by the plastic tube technique of endotherapy. (*See* vagina.)

c. *Results:* See chapter on carcinoma of the vagina.

PROSTATE

Brachytherapy for carcinoma of the prostate has been the subject of numerous trials of radiocolloidal injections (Flocks). Gold 198 seeds have also been used to treat this disease. The impossibility of establishing a target volume by direct access, the inherent dosimetric difficulties when using isolated and imbedded sources and finally the good results obtained with teletherapy (Bagshaw), has led us to conclude that brachytherapy is contraindicated in the treatment of carcinoma of the prostate and the prostatic urethra.

URINARY BLADDER

a. Clinical Anatomical Review: The urinary bladder is like a small balloon. Its walls are relatively free, except inferiorly and posteriorly where the trigone of the bladder is adherent to the floor of the pelvis. Carcinomas of the urinary bladder, especially epidermoid carcinomas, are justifiably treated with brachytherapy when they are small, that is less than 5 cm in their greatest dimension, and when they show little infiltration. Small lesions which infiltrate the musculature are also accessible to endotherapy, but more extensive lesions are more difficult to reach.

b. Recommended Technique: We recommend either the plastic tube or silk suture technique of endotherapy, accomplished at the time of the surgical intervention, under general anesthesia.

After a suprapubic cystostomy, the region of the tumor is identified and a resection of the fungating portion of the lesion is carried out leaving only its base to be implanted. A partial cystectomy is, at times, necessary if the tumor is large.

Using a curved needle, appropriate to the anatomical conditions and dimensions of the target volume, the location of each radioactive source is established by passing the needle through the muscular layers of the bladder, bringing the point of the curved needle through the bladder mucosa at the opposite side of the target volume. The corresponding plastic tube is then introduced forcefully over the point of the needle. The needle is then extracted carrying with it the plastic tube which replaces it in the bladder wall. Each plastic tube is left long enough so that it can be brought out through the cystostomy opening.

The spacing between the tubes is determined by the thickness of the target volume. It can vary between 1 and 2 cm.

The proper spacing between the tubes is further checked after releasing the retractors of the cystostomy. If necessary, a small balloon can be placed in the bladder and moderately inflated to maintain a normal size. The surgeon then closes the bladder and the skin, leaving only a very small cystostomy opening.

The dosimetry and the insertion of the Iridium 192 wires are carried out according to the usual technique (Figure 75 & 76).

Following treatment, a moderate cystitis becomes apparent in 3 to 4 weeks, while the small holes left by the plastic tubes in the cystostomy heal normally.

c. Results: Numerous techniques of brachytherapy have been advocated for the treatment of tumors of the urinary bladder. Endotherapy with radium needles and Tantalum 182 pins[2] have been used in the past. In our experience, they are less adaptable to the curved walls of the urinary bladder, which makes the plastic tube technique so advantageous. Between 1968 and 1975, we treated 23 carcinomas of the bladder. Sixteen were T_1 lesions; the remainder, T_2. Only three local recurrences have been seen (2 T_1 and 1 T_2). There were no complications. Our impression is that this technique is especially effective for small tumors less than 3 cm in diameter which do not infiltrate deeply into the bladder wall.

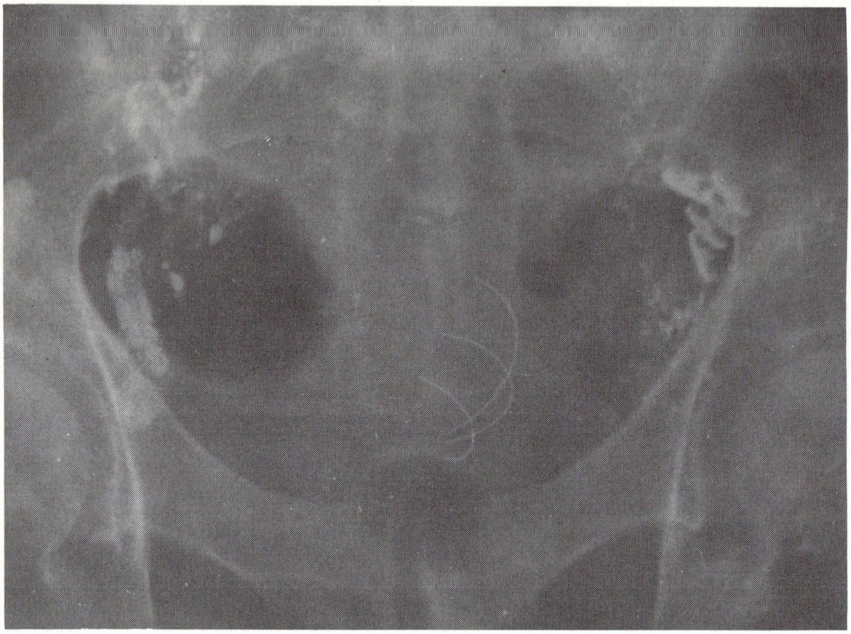

Figure 75. Cancer of the Bladder.
Plastic tube technique via suprapubic cystostomy. 3 radioactive lines.
a. Frontal roentgenogram.

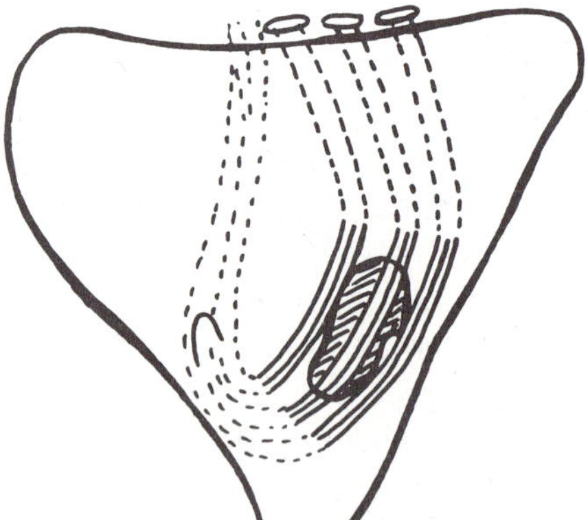

Figure 75.
b. Diagram showing relationship of sources to base of resected tumor (shaded area).

Chapter XII

MISCELLANEOUS

EMBRYONAL SARCOMAS IN CHILDREN

These are usually large poorly delimited tumors which are not amenable to implantation. However, in some instances, a proper implantation is possible; and in these cases, brachytherapy is well indicated in view of the good results obtained.

The tumors most suitable for implantation are those of the face, which do not involve bone, those of the limbs, and in a few instances, those of the pelvic region, particularly sarcoma botryoides.

All histological types of embryonal sarcomas have been treated, but the alveolar rhabdomyosarcoma of Ripelle is most often treated in view of the frequent occurrance of this pathological variety in the nasal region, which is very accessible to implantation. We recommend the plastic tube technique that can be adapted to any target volume. Single or two plane implants are used depending on the thickness of the tumor.

In cases of sarcoma botryoides of the vagina, a mold technique with Iridium 192 wires is possible, even in infant girls. This technique allows exact localization of the tumor by directly visualizing its outline on the vaginal impression. We do not recommend the use of Cesium 137 in these cases.

The dose is always high, being between 6000 and 6500 rads, given in 5 to 6 days and calculated on the reference isodose.

Adjuvant treatment is either by surgery with the implantation following the surgical procedure, or chemotherapy, or both. External radiotherapy is used in some cases to treat the associated regional lymph node areas, especially in head and neck primaries.

Results: From 1963 to 1971, 109 cases of embryonal sarcoma have been treated in the pediatric oncologic unit. Twenty of these were considered suitable for brachytherapy, 16 of the 20 are alive and well at more than one year, 5 for more than five years.

The sequellae of this treatment are surprisingly minimal; the tolerance of children to brachytherapy is particularly good.

REFERENCE

1. Chassagne, D.: Place et résultats de la curiethérapie par fils d'Iridium 192 dans 20 cas de sarcomes embryonnaires, Communications à la société Intérnationale d' oncologie. Mayence, 1971.

INDEX

D